Gary Scheiner, MS, CDE, and
Diane Herbert, MSS, LSW, CFM, CDE

– Diabetes –
How to Help

Your Complete Guide
to Caring for a Loved One
with Diabetes

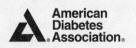

**American
Diabetes
Association.**

Associate Publisher, Books, Abe Ogden; *Director, Book Operations,* Victor Van Beuren; *Managing Editor, Books,* John Clark; *Associate Director, Book Marketing,* Annette Reape; *Acquisitions Editor,* Jaclyn Konich; *Senior Manager, Book Editing,* Lauren Wilson; *Project Manager,* Wendy Martin-Shuma; *Composition,* Circle Graphics, Inc.; *Cover Design,* Vis-à-Vis Creative Concepts; *Printer,* Versa Press.

Printed in the United States of America
1 3 5 7 9 10 8 6 4 2

The suggestions and information contained in this publication are generally consistent with the *Standards of Medical Care in Diabetes* and other policies of the American Diabetes Association, but they do not represent the policy or position of the Association or any of its boards or committees. Reasonable steps have been taken to ensure the accuracy of the information presented. However, the American Diabetes Association cannot ensure the safety or efficacy of any product or service described in this publication. Individuals are advised to consult a physician or other appropriate health care professional before undertaking any diet or exercise program or taking any medication referred to in this publication. Professionals must use and apply their own professional judgment, experience, and training and should not rely solely on the information contained in this publication before prescribing any diet, exercise, or medication. The American Diabetes Association— its officers, directors, employees, volunteers, and members—assumes no responsibility or liability for personal or other injury, loss, or damage that may result from the suggestions or information in this publication.

⊗ The paper in this publication meets the requirements of the ANSI Standard Z39.48-1992 (permanence of paper).

ADA titles may be purchased for business or promotional use or for special sales. To purchase more than 50 copies of this book at a discount, or for custom editions of this book with your logo, contact the American Diabetes Association at the address below or at booksales@diabetes.org.

American Diabetes Association
2451 Crystal Drive, Suite 900
Arlington, VA 22202

DOI: 10.2337/9781580406635

Library of Congress Cataloging-in-Publication Data

Names: Scheiner, Gary, author. | Herbert, Diane, author.
Title: Diabetes-how to help : your complete guide to caring for a loved one with diabetes / Gary Scheiner, Diane Herbert.
Description: Arlington : American Diabetes Association, [2017]
Identifiers: LCCN 2016058346 | ISBN 9781580406635
Subjects: LCSH: Diabetes--Patients--Care. | Diabetes--Patients--Family relationships. | Caregivers.
Classification: LCC RC521 .S34 2017 | DDC 616.4/62--dc23
LC record available at https://lccn.loc.gov/2016058346

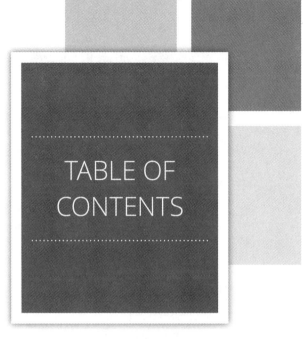

TABLE OF CONTENTS

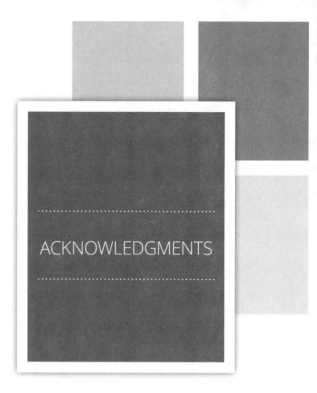

ACKNOWLEDGMENTS

Coming from someone who lives with diabetes (Gary) and someone who cares very much for someone with diabetes (Diane), thank you for taking an interest in being a better support person. It truly takes a village to manage diabetes, and we're so grateful to have you as part of the village!

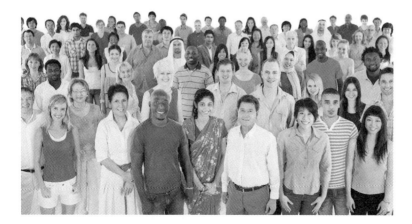

Gary thanks his wife Debbie for putting up with his high and low glucose–induced mood swings over the past 30 years and for supplying enough middle-of-the-night rapid-acting carbs to feed a small nation.

Diane sends a special thanks to her daughter Lauren, son Jackson, and husband Bob, who shared their personal experiences, attended countless conferences and discussions on diabetes, and helped her create the time to work on "the book." Diane also thanks Gary for giving her the opportunity to bring the emotional aspects of life with diabetes to the forefront.

ABOUT THE AUTHORS

Gary Scheiner, MS, CDE, is owner and clinical director of Integrated Diabetes Services (www.integrated diabetes.com), a practice located just outside of Philadelphia specializing in intensive insulin therapy and advanced education for children and adults. He and his team offer diabetes management consultations worldwide via phone and the Internet.

Gary has been a certified diabetes educator since 1995 and has managed to live an active, productive life with type 1 diabetes since he was a freshman in college. He has written six books, including *Think Like a Pancreas: A Practical Guide to Managing Diabetes with Insulin.* Gary lectures nationally and internationally for people with diabetes and was named 2014 Diabetes Educator of the Year by the American Association of Diabetes Educators. In addition to serving on the faculty of Children With Diabetes and the board of directors for the JDRF, Gary volunteers for the American Diabetes Association, DiabetesSisters, and Setebaid diabetes camps.

Gary earned a Bachelor of Arts in Psychology from Washington University in St. Louis and a Master of Science in Exercise Physiology from Benedictine University. He has been happily married to his college sweetheart, Debbie, since 1989 and has four wonderful kids: Marley, Jackie, Benjamin, and Nalani. A fitness fanatic, Gary enjoys playing basketball, running, cycling, strength training, and cheering on his Philadelphia sports teams.

Diane Herbert, MSS, LSW, CFM, CDE, and her family became directly involved with diabetes when her son was diagnosed with type 1 diabetes on his fifth birthday. Since that time, Diane has worked with families, individuals, schools, and companies to address the emotional and psychological aspects of life with diabetes to increase the understanding and overall quality of care and support for people with diabetes.

Diane is a licensed medical social worker, certified family mediator, and certified diabetes educator. Before her clinical work, Diane held executive positions in business development, strategy, and program management. Currently, Diane serves as vice president of clinical services for Livongo Health, a consumer digital health company that empowers people with chronic conditions. She maintains a private clinical practice focused on adolescents and families living with type 1 diabetes and is an advocate for people living with diabetes. She is a frequent JDRF and industry speaker and author on topics related to diabetes and child development, transition of care, and the intersection of emotional health and diabetes management.

Diane received her master's degree in Social Science from Bryn Mawr College and her bachelor's degree in Public Relations and Political Science from Virginia Polytechnic Institute

& State University, with internships at Integrated Diabetes Services, The Children's Hospital of Philadelphia, and Bryn Mawr Hospital. Diane currently serves on the advisory board of Penn Diabetes: University of Pennsylvania Health System. Diane is a clean-food foodie, newly formed tennis enthusiast, and hopeless nature and animal lover. She lives in Devon, Pennsylvania, with her husband, Bob; their kids Lauren and Jackson (type 1); and their dogs Pippa and Zeke.

Recognizing that comprehensive and effective diabetes management requires specialization in many areas, Diane and Gary work together to offer physiological and emotional support and education to improve the health and well-being of people living with diabetes.

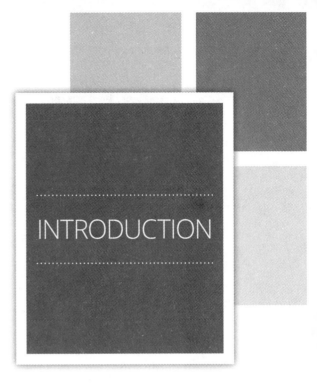

INTRODUCTION

I f you're reading this, chances are that someone close to you has diabetes. This person might be your spouse, partner, parent, child, or a special friend or relative. Even though your actions are inspired by love, dealing with someone else's diabetes can evoke a variety of unpleasant thoughts, questions, and emotions:

Should I let him eat that, or should I say something?

What if her blood glucose gets too low?
Then what do I do?

If things keep going on like this, he'll probably go blind
or lose a leg.

Why won't he just get up and move around?

This is a fine example she is setting.

Maybe I should be more involved in his diabetes.

Maybe I should be less involved in his diabetes.

I wish I understood this better so that I could do something about it.

This book is all about empowering you, the support person, to be the best support person you can be. These pages will give you a greater understanding of diabetes: what it is, what causes it, and how to manage it. You'll understand things from the standpoint of the person with diabetes and recognize the role that you play on a daily basis as well as in special situations. You'll learn when to step in and when to step back and will learn how to deal effectively with crises, both large and small. You'll also discover that you are not alone in your role as a support person. There are resources just for you, and there are strategies that can help you to take proper care of yourself while caring for someone with diabetes.

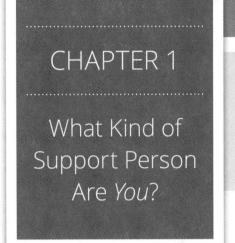

CHAPTER 1

What Kind of Support Person Are *You?*

When it comes to diabetes and loved ones, you've probably found yourself asking, "How can I help?" This book will give you tips on how to help in many areas, from the kitchen to the doctor's office, and will give you guidance on how to help your loved one emotionally as well as physically. But just as important as helping your loved one, you will learn how to help yourself. Some information will apply equally to everyone, while other information will be specific to certain types of relationships.

For Spouses and Partners

Maybe your partner had diabetes when you met, or maybe he or she was diagnosed sometime during your life together. Either way, being a partner to a person with diabetes presents a number of unique challenges.

How Do You View Your Role In Your Partner's Diabetes?

➤ Diabetes is something that belongs only to your partner.

➤ You've taken diabetes on fully as if you were diagnosed yourself.

➤ Diabetes? What diabetes?

Truth and trouble rest in each of these philosophies about the role a spouse or partner plays in living with a person with diabetes. The truth is, diabetes and diabetes management do ultimately belong to people with diabetes. Only they can decide how they feel about living with diabetes and how they are going to manage it. But as you'll learn throughout the book, diabetes is also a family affair. And whether you invite it in or not, diabetes will play a role in your relationship with your partner or spouse.

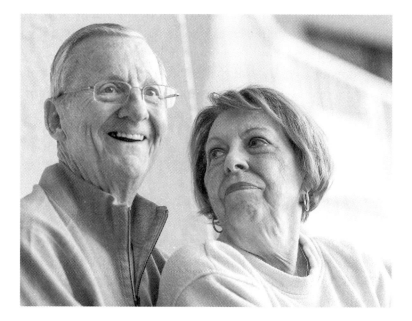

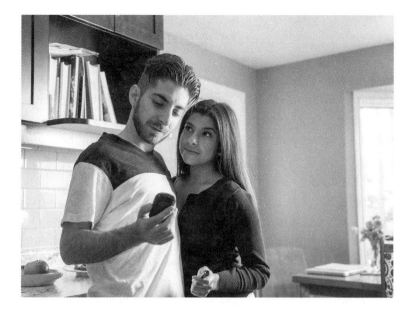

If you are living under the "Diabetes? What diabetes?" philosophy, then there's a good chance your partner with diabetes gave you this book as a not-so-subtle hint that it's important that you have some grasp of this part of his or her life. Diabetes doesn't define your partner, but it is a part of everyday life for them. Any lack of understanding, appreciation, or involvement can limit your intimacy and connection with your partner.

As with most things in life, the quest is for balance. Helping you find the balance between involvement and respecting your partner as an independent adult is the goal of this book. There are powerful and impactful ways that you can support your partner. By equipping yourself with knowledge, strategies, and tips, you will be ready to be a part of diabetes in a constructive and effective way. Sections of this book that you might find particularly helpful are: Communication and Support (page 109), Sexual Intimacy (page 168), Nutrition Fundamentals (page 134), Hypoglycemia (Low Blood Glucose) (page 181), and Piecing Together the Insurance Puzzle (page 128).

....

For Parents

To cover all the emotional, physical, practical, and tactical ways that diabetes touches your relationship with your child and your family could be a separate book entirely. Here, we start by giving you specific and necessary information and resources that you can use every day.

Although we're presenting information in the context of diabetes, the points covered are really about building understanding, communication, and tactical parenting strategies to address issues specific to raising a child. These points are helpful in the context of diabetes but will also enhance your overall relationship with your child.

In addition to the knowledge and facts about diabetes that you need, we also provide constructive ways to cope with the unique sadness, fear, and grief that you may feel as a result of your child living with diabetes. If you're at the beginning of this journey, these feelings may be compounded by a sense of feeling overwhelmed and alone.

You are not alone in this journey. There are extensive resources and connections that can help get you and your family on the path to your "new normal."

Here's a personal note from Diane sharing how she felt, and sometimes still feels, regarding her son and his diagnosis with diabetes.

> ***How do you keep it together*** *when your baby, your firstborn, gets diagnosed with diabetes on his fifth birthday? How do you get him to follow you on the journey to find a new normal when the road for as far as you can see is crowded with injections, finger pricks, doctors, hospitals, and uncertainty? How do you get him to take a road to a place where icons of happiness—birthday cake, lollipops, and ice cream— evoke fear and panic.*

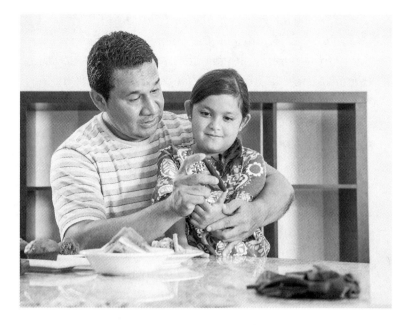

Your desire to run screaming the other way couldn't be greater, so how can you possibly convince that little boy with fearful eyes that this is the right journey to take and that he must start that journey RIGHT NOW—no warmup!

I want to bring some wisdom, magic trick, or tried-and-true answer to this question to give new parents of children with type 1 diabetes a "step by step" to surviving the crossover from life as you knew it, to life as it will forever be in the foreseeable future. I wish I could, but I really can't.

You can do this because you have strength in places you haven't yet looked. You have the love for your child that will drive you to find the way to coach him to have the confidence to manage and thrive in his new world. So you begin. You take turns with your partner staying with him in the hospital room until you can manage to wall up your own fears and emotions for today.

You dare to let yourself glimpse into the future and you realize that things that you once worried about for your kids—happiness, school, friends, safety—just hit a multiplier that would challenge the strongest math mind. You pray that the bond between you can make the monumental leap from, "Trust me, you'll love pre-school" to "Trust me, those giant needles won't hurt."

This is an endurance event. Your child must trust you. Tricks, bribes, and lollipop rewards won't get this done. Finally the question comes: "Why are we here, Mom? I want to go home." Somehow you weave together an explanation in words that you hope will reduce his panic, with words that create positive, strong images for you both.

You tell him that you've just been given orders to start an important mission to go on a science adventure to learn about our bodies. You use words like "power boosters," "clickers," "special snack," and "good stuff" to lessen the terrifying world of injections, finger pricks, and blood. But mostly, you just start moving.

You move past the comments of the uninformed. You learn to master the art of the smile and nod as good-meaning people tell you that your child's diabetes management will become as routine as brushing teeth.

You move on to your "new normal" with a positive and calm demeanor because you know he is watching your every move and taking his cues on how to handle all the unknowns from how you are handling them. You package up your own fear, worries, and sadness and save it up for night or for your brief times alone in the car.

So 6 months in, I'm definitely not going to tell you that it's just like brushing teeth, but I will tell you that our son understands the difference between strong and weak food and the importance of "listening to your body." He knows how to check his blood, he knows which numbers are "in the range" and which are high, and of course he knows which numbers mean "special snack"! He proudly wears his diabetes wristband and openly talks about it with his friends. He accepts the fact that we check blood six to eight times a day and that eating means injections. And if you ask him, above all, he's counting the days until he gets his very own diabetic alert dog (as of today, his name will be Barky).

Diabetes is a family affair, and while the fact that my son's childhood has been colored by this condition makes me sad in ways that are difficult to put into words, it has also brought a strength and bond to our family that gives me the peace to know we are able to handle our future. Diabetes is a part of us, but it is not the soul of us.

You can do this! You are in the company of tens of thousands of amazing parents of kids with diabetes and kids who teach us grace and resilience. And, above all, these kids show us that life goes on.

Transition of Care

The term "transition of care" usually refers to shifting from one care provider to another. For the purposes of this book, transition of care is about shifting diabetes management responsibility from the caregiver to the person with diabetes (i.e., from parent to child). The journey from parent-provided care to self-care can be full of challenges and potholes. But it can also give you a reason to have a purposeful approach to parenting and clear communication with your child. Having a roadmap and plan can help avoid some common obstacles as well as give you strategies to get past challenges when they do arise.

What can make this transition process so challenging? To name a few things, the desire for independence; the desire to fit in with peers; hectic, varied schedules; fluctuating hormone levels; worry and anxiety; multiple caregivers; and varied and nonlinear stages of development are all reasons. Clearly, there are many factors that add to the complexity of managing diabetes as a child grows. To begin with, there are no hard and fast rules on when kids should start taking over various parts of their diabetes care. With all aspects of development, kids reach emotional and physical milestones at various times. These guidelines and factors give you things to consider to help build a smooth(er) transition for you and your child.

Many issues can be avoided if you go in with a clear distinction between diabetes *skill level* and diabetes *maturity level*. Kids are smart and capable learners and will surprise you with how quickly they can learn and master diabetes skills—especially ones that use technology! Skills like performing blood glucose checks, giving injections, treating a low, or operating insulin pumps are often learned at a fairly early age.

But wait! Having the *ability* to do something like checking blood glucose or giving an insulin injection and having the *maturity* to remember (or to stop doing something fun) to do them are two vastly different things. Depending on the age of your child and when he or she was diagnosed with diabetes, there could be many years between these two stages.

My Kid Is Only 3: I've Got Time

Transition of care actually begins at diagnosis. Even if your child is too young to take on any diabetes care tasks directly, an important part of transition of care still takes place. Right out of the gate, your approach to diabetes management lays the foundation for how your child will approach diabetes management for years to come. Here are things you can do at any age, to pave the way for successful adoption of diabetes self-management down the road.

Create the Mood

Our kids take their cues from us. If we're anxious and nervous about diabetes, it's likely that they will be too. However, if you're calm and confident, your child will likely follow your lead. Whenever possible, take emotions out of diabetes management tasks. View them as routine, nonnegotiable parts of the day. Sometimes things will go according to plan and many times they will not. Try to approach both situations with discipline—sort of like a coach who doesn't get too overjoyed when the team wins, or too upset when they lose. Instead, the coach gives encouragement and support for playing the game. A good coach can highlight things that you did well, talk about opportunities for improvement, and help make a plan for the next game. Taking a coaching approach to diabetes management helps reduce everyone's apprehension, guilt, and anxiety.

Create routines that communicate to your child that diabetes management is a priority, even when other things are going on. At the same time, you can demonstrate that diabetes management tasks don't require a great deal of excitement or drama, even when things don't go according to plan.

• • ☐ **TIP:** Keep your focus on the *management* aspect of diabetes versus the potential consequences of diabetes. This shift in focus empowers you to know that you are able to handle whatever comes your way. Kids will pick up on your feelings of empowerment and as a result are likely to feel more secure and empowered to manage diabetes as well.

Take a look at an example of two different ways that our energy can be directed.

Let's say your daughter checks her blood glucose and it's 38 mg/dL. Having a blood glucose of 38 is an energy-packed situation. An energetic response is actually appropriate and helpful since a low blood glucose reading requires action and a sense of urgency. So the question becomes, how do we use that energy constructively?

With our focus on "How do I manage this situation?" your energy goes toward treating the blood glucose by getting and giving your daughter a source of fast-acting sugar. By contrast, if you focus instead on what could have happened if you didn't check her blood or what would happen if she doesn't eat something right away, then your demeanor, tone, and reaction all become fear-based.

If energy from the low blood glucose is allowed to feed fear and anxiety, people often find themselves reacting with statements like, "How did you let your blood sugar get so low?" or "How did I let this happen?" or "Oh my gosh; you're 38! Drink this, drink this . . . now!" This response makes the situation stressful and anxious for everyone and distracts from the goal of getting everyone working together to treat the low blood glucose.

If reactions continue to be emotionally charged with fear and anxiety, over time, the child's response to a low blood glucose reading may be one of anxiety. Kids may start to believe, "I'm bad if my blood glucose goes low," "Mommy gets mad at me when my blood glucose goes low," or "Something is really wrong with me, and I'm not safe if I'm not with Mommy or Daddy."

In turn, these thoughts lead to behaviors like not wanting to check blood glucose levels or not wanting to spend time away from parents. Low blood glucose levels are going to happen. Your goal as caregiver is to remove judgment from the person (this includes yourself) and focus your energy on treating the blood glucose. The message we want to impart to our kids is that they (and you!) have the knowledge and the tools needed to manage diabetes—even the worrisome parts like low blood glucose levels. This message doesn't change the reality of diabetes, but it does empower you and your loved ones with diabetes to handle life with diabetes.

Verbalize Diabetes Management Tasks

If there can be an upside to diabetes management and the process of teaching kids about self-care, it's the fact that you have the chance for practice. Lots of practice. And of course we all know practice makes better. Notice we didn't say perfect—just better!

Verbalizing tasks with kids starts them on their way to learning what they need to know. Talk through blood glucose readings: "Your blood glucose is 65. That's below target. We need to treat that with some fast sugar." As they get a little older, you could say, "Your blood glucose is 65. Is that above, below, or in your target zone?" and then "Your blood glucose is 65. What do you think we need to do?"

You can build progressively more advanced conversations about carb counting, insulin calculations, treating high and low blood glucose levels, how your child feels when glucose levels are high or low, food choices, and activity planning. Make these conversations part of your routine and have fun with them. Adding a game element such as "guess how many carbs" or "high, low, in the zone" makes learning more fun and helps concepts stick.

Look for opportunities to give your child knowledge in ways that aren't scary or overly emotional. You don't need to approach diabetes education as "you have to learn this because your life depends on it!" Simply using a matter-of-fact, nonnegotiable approach will let your child know that diabetes management is serious. Scare tactics typically work against you in the long run.

Answer Questions Honestly

Without facts, kids will fill in the blanks on their own. And often, they will fill them in with incorrect or incomplete information. Whether you're ready or not, kids will pick up bits and pieces of the "diabetes big picture" and make their own connections where facts are missing. As difficult as it may be, when kids ask questions, even ones you don't think they're ready to handle, it's important to give an age-appropriate, accurate answer.

Here are some tough questions that your child will likely ask at some point and some answers that you can use as a guide to think about how you would answer. In general, your response should factor in your child's age and maturity level. The younger the child is, the fewer details he or she will need to be satisfied. Also, think about your child's personality. Does he like statistics and facts? Does she find comfort in talking things through? Factoring in these preferences will help you prepare for difficult conversations. Remember when we said that diabetes will help you with other areas of your parent-child relationship? Well, getting practice with difficult conversations about diabetes will help you and your child with future discussions about other topics parents worry about, such as driving, alcohol or drug use, and sex.

Sample Difficult Questions

CHILD "Dad, am I going to have diabetes forever?"

YOU "I'm not 100% sure. The scientists are working really hard, all the time, to find a way to make it go away, but they haven't found the answer yet."

This would be an example of how to answer a young child. As your child gets older, you would build in additional information about the types of research efforts and where they are in the process and provide ways for your child to get involved through groups like the Juvenile Diabetes Research Foundation (JDRF) and others.

CHILD "Dad, can you die from diabetes?"

YOU "Yes, we can die from many things, including diabetes. That's why we do things to give our body what it needs to be healthy, like take insulin and eat healthy foods. It's also why we do things like wear a helmet and hold hands crossing the street—to help protect our bodies."

Adding the non-diabetes realities of risks we face helps the child neutralize the feeling that he or she is less safe than others. For older children, you would discuss the specific aspects of diabetes that can cause death or other complications while explaining how keeping blood glucose levels in target range as much as possible reduces risks. This approach gives children the understanding that they have a great deal of control over what happens.

CHILD "What happens if I have a low blood glucose and you're not there?"

PARENT "I've talked to your teachers and your school nurse about diabetes and low blood glucose levels. They know what to do and will help you if you have a low blood glucose reaction while I'm away. Be sure to tell them if you're not feeling well or think you might be low. Also remember you have a juice box in your desk."

Here you're starting the transition that tells the child that other adults besides their parents can help them, but also that they can help themselves.

Helping children troubleshoot their fears is a powerful way to support their ability to gain confidence in diabetes management. Even if your child isn't coming to you with these types of questions, that doesn't mean he or she isn't thinking about them. These situations are important to role-play and discuss. Some kids think about potential situations more than you'd like, and others won't think about them at all until they are in the middle of one. For those kids, it's good for the parents to get the conversation started by asking something like "What would you do if your blood glucose went low while you were at school?" Kids benefit from having honest answers combined with information that helps them feel able to handle the truth rather than feeling helpless or fearful of the unknown.

Model a Healthy Lifestyle

A healthy lifestyle for people with diabetes is the same as it is for someone who doesn't have diabetes (discussed in detail in Chapter 5). Eat healthy, get regular exercise, and find ways to manage stress. Sound familiar? When you choose healthy foods in appropriate portions, make physical activity a priority, and find ways to handle stress constructively, you greatly increase the chances that your kids will adopt similar habits.

For example, setting a tone in the family that distinguishes foods and activities that happen on vacation or at special occasions from our regular routines and habits is a good way to teach balance. French fries don't have to be forbidden, but it's not healthy to include them at every meal. Having an alcoholic drink to celebrate with friends or at the end of the week is different than using alcohol to deal with stress.

Whether kids push a pretend mower behind you while you mow the lawn or pretend to be going to work, they are modeling our behaviors. Consider making healthy lifestyle choices a chance to get a two-for-one. You'll be healthier and feel better and your child will have a foundation of healthy habits!

It's Time for Your Child to Self-Manage: You've Got This!
When is the right time for kids and teens to "self-manage" diabetes? The answer is as clear as mud. As with all learning, each child will develop and progress at his or her own pace. Factors that influence when your child will be ready to take on aspects of diabetes management will depend on your child's individual maturity level, personality, age at diagnosis, and his or her home situation. The table below provides general guidance for transitioning kids' ownership of various types of diabetes-related tasks.

Guidelines for Transitioning Kids' Ownership of Diabetes-Related Tasks

Age Range (years)	Diabetes Self-Care Stage	What It Might Look Like
0–5	Care provided by adult	Adult is fully responsible for all aspects of diabetes management
5–9	Child has some involvement and adult is there to supervise	Child checks blood glucose but adult prompts and helps to see that it's done properly
6–11	Child has responsibility for some tasks and is beginning to learn more complex ones; the adult is there to supervise	Child is responsible for morning blood glucose check, talks about insulin dosing, gives self-injections/bolus; parent confirms amounts and plan
8–12	Child has responsibility for basic tasks, and adult provides remote supervision	Child checks blood glucose, counts carbs, and gives insulin with phone or text support from adult
13–16	Teen takes primary responsibility for daily tasks, and adult provides support, accountability, and troubleshooting	Weekly joint review of glucose logs to identify patterns and needs for adjustments and to ensure tasks are being taken care of by teen
17+	Teen/young adult has ownership of diabetes management	Parents and caregivers transition to a support role

Another way to look at it is to consider the caregiver's evolving role:

- Doer
  - Doer, Educator, and Supporter
    - Sometimes Doer, Educator, Expectation Setter, Enforcer, and Supporter
      - Emergency Backup, Troubleshooter, and Supporter
        - Supporter

Many families get stuck in the "doer" phase for longer than is reasonable or appropriate. *Doing* is actually easier, faster, and less conflictual than evolving through to the other phases. We can't stress enough that one of the best gifts you can give your child with diabetes is positive support to progressively grow into owning his or her diabetes management. Recognizing this may help you resist the temptation to hold on to diabetes responsibilities for too long or to be too forgiving of a lack of accountability on your child's part.

We mentioned previously that the ability for a child to take on new tasks is highly individualized. Avoid the temptation to make transitions at arbitrary milestones: "You're 14. Diabetes is yours now." or "You're in high school. You have to do this yourself." These ages may be reasonable times for some kids to have greater ownership of diabetes, but not all and definitely not all at once.

Here are some signs in a child's development that may signal he or she is ready for additional diabetes responsibilities/ownership:

➤ **Motor and cognitive skill development:** Child is more independent with other self-care routines (dressing, brushing teeth, making bed).

➤ **Body awareness and modesty:** Child starts to have concern about being seen naked by you/others or concern about "private parts."

➤ **Confidence and independence:** This is best described as the "I got this" phase. Of course, they don't fully, but it's important to capitalize on this developmental phase and give the child increased responsibility with supervision and support.

➤ **Desire for caregiver distance:** The child wants more privacy from caregivers; he or she wants to spend time away from home, and peers gain importance.

➤ **Forced caregiver distance:** Child engages in school, camps, trips with others, or college.

If you know a milestone is coming—like camp or a sleepover—start preparing for it a few weeks or months ahead to make sure that your child will have the skills needed to participate safely and confidently. Prepare by asking:

➤ What's needed for you to feel that your child will be safe?

➤ What's needed for your child to actually be safe?

➤ What skills does your child need to be safe during this activity?

➤ Give time to educate, practice, gain confidence, and plan (hint: the night before isn't enough time).

It's hard for parents to "let go" of their children, and it can be *really* hard when your child has diabetes. But while there may be some situations that logistically just won't work (yet), especially when sleeping away from home is involved, try to work out a plan that allows kids to participate in a range of activities. A good test is to ask yourself, "Would I say 'yes' if my child didn't have diabetes?" If the answer is "yes," then start making a plan to be able to say "yes" to your child with diabetes. Your secret weapon is preparation and practice.

Knowing how kids learn at different ages can also help you build teaching methods that are most likely to be effective. For young kids, learning happens best by doing. When kids reach school-age (8–12 years old), it's time to teach. If you like to talk and explain things to your kids, now's your time to shine! By the time your kid becomes a teen, they learn best through modeling. You may have the feeling that everything you say to your teen is falling on deaf ears, because it pretty much is. Teens respond to action and modeling.

How Children Learn at Different Ages

Child's Age (years)	Learning Method	Example
0–7	Doing	Let them do tasks like check blood glucose and count carbs.
8–12	Listening, teaching	Explain the "what" and "why" of diabetes.
13–19	Modeling	Demonstrate importance of diabetes tasks by being clear and consistent. Make healthy lifestyle choices.

Failure to Launch

You'll hear us say this throughout the book—diabetes doesn't happen in a vacuum. Teen years have the reputation of being marked by hormones, rebellion, and a seemingly endless ability to ignore what parents and other adults say. If you're raising a child with diabetes, you may be either dreading the impact of these factors on diabetes management or living them.

There is good news here! Studies show that the vast majority of kids have healthy physical, cognitive, emotional, social, and sexual development through adolescent years. There are general things you can do to foster positive youth development and specific things that are essential to support your child's ability and willingness to manage his or her diabetes. Positive youth development can be fostered by focusing on the five Cs.

The Five Cs for Positive Youth Development

Trait	Definition	How to Foster
Competence	Perception that one has abilities and skills	Provide training and practice in specific skills, both academic and hands-on
Confidence	Internal sense of self-efficacy and positive self-worth	Provide opportunities for young people to experience success when trying new things
Connection	Positive bond with people and institutions	Build relationships between youth and peers, teachers, and parents
Character	A sense of right and wrong, integrity, and respect for standards of behavior	Provide opportunities to practice increasing self-control and spiritual development
Caring	A sense of sympathy and empathy for others	Care for young people

Think about applying another column to the five Cs to illustrate how this approach would be applied to the area of healthy diabetes self-care.

Trait	How to Foster Specifically for Diabetes
Competence	Teach kids about diabetes management through verbalization of tasks, gamification to reinforce fact retention, and giving them access to their health care providers and other resources.
Confidence	Transition diabetes tasks a little at a time rather than all at once.
Connection	Expose kids to community activities sponsored by organizations such as JDRF, Children With Diabetes, diabetes camps, and other organizations in your community.
Character	Stress the importance of honesty and discuss the impact of dishonesty (sneaking food can lead to dosing errors, loss of trust leads to loss of privileges).
Caring	Show empathy and understanding that diabetes is a lot of work and a real challenge.

If the diabetes management handoff isn't going so smoothly in your family, there are two likely culprits: time and guilt. These two factors can lead otherwise effective parents to feel completely at a loss for what to do to get their child to take care of his or her diabetes.

When parenting your child through the diabetes change of control, each family will have unique traditions, styles, and beliefs about parenting. However, studies show that when kids are provided with clear expectations, consistency, natural consequences, and support, they learn, grow, and succeed.

While the nuances of your child and your situation are real, things will feel less chaotic and confusing if you can bring yourself back to a few guiding principles and specific rules.

Nobody Is Going to Like Having Diabetes—Period.

As parents, we want our kids to be happy: happy at school, happy with their friends, and, believe it or not, happy with their diabetes. This want is both unrealistic and problematic. It is *unrealistic* in the sense that, yes, we can hope and expect that our kids will get through the shock and grief of diagnosis, but really who and why would anybody be *happy* about the additional burden and hassles that diabetes brings? It is *problematic* in that when our kids express dislike, anger, or sadness about diabetes, we feel bad and try to change it. We try to change it by telling ourselves, "Well, maybe if I do this for her, she won't be so upset" or "I know I told him to text me his number, but he really hates having to deal with diabetes when he's with his friends."

When Great Parents Get Bad Results

Time and guilt cloud our otherwise clear parenting minds, and all of a sudden, our parenting decisions and actions become very conflicted. You say that diabetes management is your child's responsibility, but you constantly bring the test kit when it gets forgotten, check to see if a bolus was given, take care of reviewing blood glucose logs, and make adjustments to basal rates on your own (clear expectations—gone).

Then because we feel bad that our kids have to deal with diabetes all the time, we let them off the hook for not doing what we told them to do (natural consequences—gone).

We wake up and realize the error of our ways and swear to "tighten up" all things related to diabetes management. Things get better for a little while, but then a big project comes up at work, your partner is out of town, and the dog is sick, and all of your good intentions get waylaid (consistency—gone).

Now you're looking at the blood glucose logs for the past month, and numbers are all over the place. Panic kicks in and you start yelling at your kid asking, "Why aren't you taking care of your diabetes?" "You know that you have GOT to do this!" "You need to be responsible for your care!" (support—gone).

If any of this (or all of this) sounds familiar, take heart; you're definitely not alone. Getting through transition of diabetes care in the teen years is not easy, but it is both doable and fairly straightforward. Simplistically stated, these years should include providing clear expectations, consistency, natural consequences, and support. But how do you actually carry out these actions when managing diabetes tasks in real life?

Developmentally, it's totally appropriate for diabetes to be at the very bottom of your child's priority list. If your teen is given the choice between hanging out with friends or taking care of diabetes, friends will likely win. It's the role of parents to make diabetes a nonnegotiable priority.

We already learned earlier in this section that teens don't learn through talking, lecturing, and reasoning. In fact, the part of the brain that manages executive function (decision-making) isn't fully developed until age 25, give or take a year. So adopting a parenting strategy that gives the decision-making to the teen is a bad idea (e.g., "Should I take care of my diabetes or hang with my friends?").

Having said that, the teen years also may not be the time to go for the "gold standard" of diabetes care and an A1C of 5.5%. Rather, make sure your child is accountable for self-care and is consistently doing what he or she needs to do to be healthy. Having realistic expectations about how interested or diligent your child will be at this stage will also go a long way in preserving your overall relationship. And keeping your relationship intact will greatly improve your ability to help your child navigate the difficulties of growing up, including those related to diabetes.

To help keep things simple, we've created four diabetes rules to use during the teen years.

1. **Self-care is nonnegotiable.** Here are the minimum requirements for diabetes self-care:
   - Check blood glucose a minimum of four times a day (by way of fingerstick or continuous glucose monitor)

- Take insulin *before* eating
- Carry fast-acting glucose (always)

2. **Review logs and follow communication plan (example to follow).** It seems that speed dial has completely removed our ability to remember phone numbers. That same lack of connection and account-ability are lost when we only rely on technology to capture and send our blood glucose logs. Having to regularly (weekly) review and think about numbers, trends, and patterns fosters ownership and under-standing of the numbers and sets the stage for problem-solving.

3. **You don't have to like diabetes or diabetes tasks, you just have to do them.** There are many things in life that kids don't like doing. Book reports, cleaning rooms, cleaning up after the dog, diabetes tasks—they're all responsibilities. It's okay for your kids to be mad or upset that they have to do them; in fact, it's healthy for them to share that frustration.

4. **Reframe. Diabetes misbehavior = any other form of misbehavior.** If you caught your child drinking and driving, skipping school, or lying about where they were, there would be consequences. Having a mindset that diabetes misbehavior is the same as any other misbehavior will help you set and enforce appropriate consequences and boundaries.

Putting Rules into Action

Having a written family diabetes agreement in place removes any confusion over what's expected. Once you have this plan in place and you've clearly stated what diabetes responsibil-ities your child has, step back and let your child step up. For your child, it should be a huge relief that you're only going to be asking about diabetes once a week during your designated diabetes talk time!

····· ☐ TIPS FOR SUCCESS:

- Pick a day and time when your household is usually quiet and relaxed as your time to review diabetes.

- Follow through. Without your commitment to follow through, there's no reason to go any further with this. Follow-through applies to both your child's behaviors and yours. The "win" for kids in this agreement is that they get relief from the constant stream of questions about what they did and didn't do with their diabetes care. Resist the temptation to ask until your review time. We realize this takes a huge leap of faith. But remember, just because you asked if they did something doesn't mean you're going to get a straight answer. It's better to wait for the facts (logs) and avoid the scenario where you are questioning if they are telling you the truth.

- Keep it simple. Think about the times that you really *need* to know about high and low blood glucose levels and only include those times in your plan. For example, if your child has a low at school and the school nurse can help, do you really need to know about that low at that moment?

- Don't fall for the "I forgot" line. Kids remember the lyrics to hundreds of songs and the social details and dramas of countless friends. Believe us, it's not a memory issue; it's a priority/choice issue.

Sample Family Diabetes Plan and Communication Agreement

Kids want their parents to get off their back about diabetes care. Parents are worried sick about how their child is going to manage diabetes while away from home or as they take over their own care. This communication agreement will help you create your own plan so that everyone feels more comfortable and less stressed about diabetes management.

Diabetes Self-Care Goals (write your own; this is only an example)

For the person with diabetes:

1. Maintain blood glucose levels in the target range 70% of the time

2. Be able to spend time away from home

3. Have freedom from a constant barrage of questions and accusations about diabetes management

For the person living with a loved one with diabetes:

1. Have peace of mind that the person with diabetes is safe and taking the necessary steps to maintain good health most of the time

Diabetes Self-Care Goals

I promise to . . .	If you promise to . . .
1. Check my blood glucose *X* times/day	1. Not ask me what my glucose is
2. Bolus **before** eating	2. Not ask me if I bolused
3. Carry supplies to treat a low	3. Let me out of your sight
4. Check my blood glucose before driving	4. Let me use the car from time to time

Other Ideas to Incorporate

➤ Communication: When/how will you check in? How often?

➤ Frequency of blood glucose log discussions: how often, what will be discussed

  ▪ Recommend to start with a weekly review of blood glucose readings to identify trends and jointly problem-solve any situations/times of day when levels are consistently out of range.

- Also talk about performance and any privileges earned or lost (consequences), e.g., if a teen living with diabetes wants to go directly to a friend's house after school, to earn this privilege, he needs to demonstrate 2 weeks of glucose checks at dismissal and text results to parents.

➤ High/low blood glucose action plan (map out the expectation for each, e.g., if your blood glucose is higher than 180 mg/dL, give correction bolus)

➤ Wearing medical ID

➤ Set changes if on a pump (frequency)

➤ Rotation of sites (injection/infusion)

Once you and your child have *jointly* developed a diabetes care plan including goals, actions, and communication parameters, it's critical that you clearly identify and document the consequences if the plan isn't followed. Ideally, consequences are aligned with privileges and these consequences are clear and enforced by all caregivers. Each of your promise statements should have a consequence if broken.

Sample Promise Statements and Consequences

Privilege	Responsibility	Consequence
Going to friend's house	Check and text blood glucose at stated time	No going to friend's house for X days
Driving	Check blood glucose before driving	No driving for X days

For parents, the distinction between support and "doing" can seem muddy at times. Depending on the age of your child, he or she may not be able to perform self-care. The principle mapped out above is still the same. For children growing up with diabetes, gaining confidence is a key piece to their ability to take on diabetes management for themselves and develop a sense of independence. They gain this confidence by gradually increasing their role in diabetes management and by being supported in their ability to learn from mistakes and new situations.

Case in point: As parents, we support our children in learning to eat. At first, we feed them; then we let them try to feed themselves (but we're there making sure that they eat). They won't do it well at first, but with practice and positive reinforcement, they will gradually gain the skills they need to do it on their own. Eventually, they feed themselves. At no time during this journey are we viewing our kids as sick or incapable. And because we don't view them as incapable of feeding themselves, *they* don't feel like they are incapable of feeding themselves.

We'll go deeper into this in the section on importance of word choice and reframing, but this concept directly translates to how *supporting* a person with diabetes is very different than *taking care of* a person with diabetes. For kids, the goal is to align developmentally appropriate diabetes tasks with your child's roles/responsibilities in diabetes care. If from the very start we perceive and treat diabetes tasks the same way we do other development paths (e.g., learning to eat), they are more likely to develop a sense of confidence and empowerment.

....

For Siblings

Whether you're young or old (or in between), living life as a sibling to a person with diabetes brings many unique, important, and often-overlooked challenges and emotions.

Your relationship with your brother or sister is likely the longest relationship you will have in your lifetime.

You know each other closely as kids, as teens, as adults, and in old age. The amount of time you and your sibling are going to know each other is reason enough to do what you can to foster a loving and supportive relationship. Acknowledging this special relationship doesn't always prevent you from driving each other crazy at times and viewing the world in dramatically different ways!

Let's first talk about what it feels like to be the one *without* diabetes; the one whose needs often come second; the one who, when sick with the flu, is seen as "he'll be fine, no big deal"; the one who worries about his sister in the middle of the night when he hears their parents get up for juice boxes; the one who gets dragged to doctor appointments but doesn't get the prize afterwards; the one who gets asked to make sure his sister does what she is supposed to do; the one who worries that maybe you'll get diabetes too; or the one who lives with parents who are exhausted and stressed from caring for

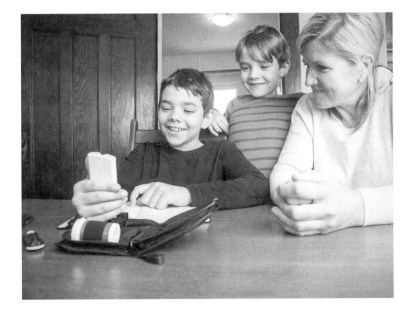

a child with diabetes. Your sibling may have diabetes, but make no mistake, you definitely have lived with it.

Your love for your sibling has brought you to this book, and your brother or sister is very lucky to have you. You can provide your sibling with a type of support that's powerful and special. Because you're probably close in age, you have an inside view of what it's like for your sibling at school, what it's like on the sports field, or what it's like to live with *your* parents. The two of you may share things with each other that you don't want to share with your parents or other adults. All of this intimate, historic, and current knowledge helps you read when your sibling is feeling down or frustrated, when he or she is making poor decisions, when he or she needs your help, and when it's time to ask for outside help.

In addition to learning the facts and how-to about diabetes (see Chapter 2), be sure to spend time on the sections talking about taking care of yourself (see Hello—What About You? and Strategies to Combat Caregiver Fatigue in Chapter 3). In fact, consider reading the section on self-care first before digging into the diabetes sections.

A Special Note for Siblings

Make sure your needs are being met and your voice is being heard. You don't have diabetes but you have struggles and challenges of your own, you need support and encouragement from your family to pursue your interests, and you need for people to check in with you from time to time to see how you're feeling. Speak up and let your family know what you need; they love you very much and will be glad you did.

A Special Note for Parents

We know your plate is full, and sometimes it's easy to lose sight of the fact that your child(ren) without diabetes feel much of the stress and worry that you feel about living with diabetes in the family. They also have their own needs that, on the surface, may seem petty compared to life with diabetes, but their needs aren't petty. Take time to balance your attention and energy and help them feel comfortable talking about their feelings.

Young siblings may respond to life with diabetes in one of two ways. They may resent the sibling with diabetes and act out to gain the attention they feel they are missing. Or they may become (or be) parentified and feel responsible for their sibling and guilty about ever asking for what they need.

In either scenario, the best approach is to validate your child's feelings and avoid making comparisons between his or her complaints and problems and what it's like to have diabetes.

It may be tempting to tell siblings who are complaining that "Sam and his stupid diabetes gets all the attention" that they should be happy that they don't have diabetes and that they don't have to get shots, but this is not a fair statement.

It's definitely challenging to be fair when one child is crying because they don't want a shot or don't want to do a site change and your other child is crying because he has to miss his favorite TV show. But disappointment and anger are being experienced by both kids. Offering both kids validation for their feelings, e.g., "I understand that you're mad and upset—I would be too!" will go a long way to reduce their need to escalate their reactions to get the support they need.

Communication, empowering siblings with knowledge, and providing age-appropriate ways to contribute to diabetes management are all effective ways to minimize the negative impact diabetes can have on family relationships. In fact, a shared family experience and mission can create powerful and lasting family bonds—even when the root is something like diabetes.

Be Your Sibling's Wingman

Siblings, you have the unique ability to be a "wingman" to your brother or sister. By this, we mean that within 1 year after diagnosis, you likely have learned a great deal about your sibling's diabetes. You've learned the areas in which your sibling excels, the areas where he or she struggles, and the friction points at home regarding diabetes management. This knowledge, combined with how well you know your brother or sister, is a powerful combination when it comes to being able to help.

In no way are you responsible for taking care of your brother or sister's diabetes. But you're in the inner circle of family, and here are some things you can do to support your sibling.

Listen

Recognize that your sibling's frustration and anger about diabetes will be greater at certain times in life than others, e.g., in new social situations, with increased responsibility, or when it's time to go away from home. Offering an understanding ear and encouragement is a powerful way to show support. Your sibling may open up to you about fears or concerns if he or she isn't comfortable telling friends or parents.

Pitch In

While diabetes is not your responsibility, viewing diabetes tasks as a family affair and having a helping attitude reduces the burden that any one person has to carry. For example, the test kit has a way of always being upstairs when you need it downstairs and downstairs when you need it upstairs. Be willing to make some of those trips up and down the stairs to show your sibling support and to save him or her a few steps.

Over the years, your help and support will make a real difference in how burnt-out your sibling may feel. This "pitch in" attitude can be applied to getting a juice box when needed, organizing the supply area, or running to the drugstore to pick up a prescription (provided you have your license, of course).

Do Some Legwork

Staying current with new diabetes technology, apps, prescription discount programs, insurance plans, and healthy eating resources is hugely time-consuming. It's easy to "hear" about programs and products, but it takes time to research how they really work, if your insurance will cover it, and where to get it. Taking on some of this legwork will make it easier for your sibling to take advantage of the latest diabetes tools and resources. However, before doing this research, make sure your sibling is interested in learning about the topic and that you aren't just sending a stream of unwelcome information.

How to Get Younger Siblings Involved

Parents can give younger siblings specific diabetes tasks. This process fosters the family spirit of pitching in and gives younger siblings a chance to feel like they are helping. Giving younger siblings a way to contribute reduces the anxiety that they feel about diabetes. Sometimes the child with diabetes won't want their siblings involved in his or her direct care, and this should be respected. There are still indirect ways for siblings to help that will keep them from feeling shut out while respecting the personal boundaries of the person with diabetes.

Some tasks that younger siblings can tackle:

➤ Count juice boxes or other supplies to see if they are running low.

➤ Bring test kit at mealtimes.

➤ Tell an adult if the continuous glucose monitor (CGM) alarm goes off or if the sibling says he or she feels low or is acting in a way that is consistent with low blood glucose.

For Extended Family

Thank you for reading this book! Even if you are not on the front lines of diabetes management, you play a part in setting the *life with diabetes tone* in your family.

Will Sam feel like the "special" one at family functions who "can't eat sugar"? Or will he feel that people on his home turf, his loved ones, get what diabetes *really* is and what goes into management? Will they know to offer the kind of help that is actually helpful? Reading this book gives you the tools you need to channel your love and concern for your family member with diabetes into meaningful and constructive support. Some sections that will be especially helpful are Nutrition Fundamentals (page 134), Di-a-What? (Diabetes Defined) (page 44), What's Your Diabetes Emotional Health? (page 76), and Hypoglycemia (Low Blood Glucose) (page 181).

For Friends

The buddy system is a wonderful thing! For a person with diabetes, a friend who has a basic understanding of diabetes can provide powerful emotional support and be a key part of physical safety. As friends, you share many of the social aspects of life together. You're together on the soccer field, traveling, out at parties, or in a host of other settings.

When you combine your knowledge of your friend's personality, likes, dislikes, and emotional needs with some basic understanding of diabetes care, you can make a big difference in how a person feels about living with diabetes. Diabetes care doesn't just take place in the doctor's office—it happens out in the real world, every day, with you.

You have a strong influence on your friend's emotional health and have an opportunity to offset feelings of isolation and differentness that sometimes come with living with diabetes.

Here are some simple but hugely powerful things to do for your friend with diabetes:

➤ Build in time to allow your friend to check blood glucose before eating.

➤ Make sure he or she doesn't get left behind when stopping to take care of diabetes tasks.

➤ Recognize blood glucose levels may be causing your friend to be moody, and don't take it personally.

➤ Know the symptoms of hypoglycemia (low blood sugar) and how to treat it.

➤ Be bold and call for help when needed. When in doubt, call. It's better to be safe than sorry.

The sections of the book that will be particularly useful to you are Hypoglycemia (Low Blood Glucose) (page 181), Di-a-What? (Diabetes Defined) (page 44), Nutrition Fundamentals (page 134), and Alcohol and Diabetes (page 158).

....

For Kids with a Parent Who Has Diabetes

You may not be "the parent," but as time progresses, your parent with diabetes may need you to play an increasing role in diabetes management. When your adult parent/child relationship starts to change from them parenting you to you feeling like you are parenting them, it can be an awkward situation for you both. It takes time, sensitivity, and information to successfully transition into playing a supporting role for your aging parent.

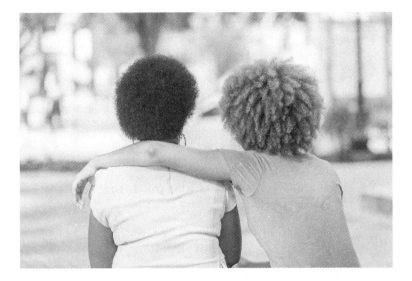

Similar to financial issues, it's important that you understand your aging parent's diabetes routines, medications, doctors, and insurance information. Diabetes management is something that changes over time, so it's a topic to revisit on a regular basis to make sure that your information is current. Talk about how you're going to share information and what support your parent needs from you now, and make plans for how this might look in the future so you can plan and identify available resources in the community.

It's likely that a great deal has changed since your parents were diagnosed. Learning to use new diabetes technology, whether it's a smartphone or an insulin pump, may not be easy for your parent. When combined with their own changes in vision, dexterity, and memory, diabetes tasks that were once "old hat" can quickly become overwhelming and difficult to maintain. Because these changes often happen gradually, it can be hard for your parent to notice or admit that he or she isn't able to do the things like before.

Working together with your parent and a health care provider, you can find ways to modify and simplify the diabetes management routine to accommodate the changes that come with age.

Some ways to modify or simplify diabetes tasks:

➤ Use meters with larger displays or talking meters.

➤ Use insulin pens that have fixed or easier dosing mechanisms.

➤ Use combination medications (meds that combine two different prescription drugs into one) to reduce the total number of pills to manage. Ask the pharmacist or physician to review all medications your parents are taking to see if the number of medications can be streamlined by combination drugs.

Prescription costs are a concern for everyone, but for a person on a fixed income, these costs can be a barrier to being healthy and being able to take medications as prescribed by the doctor. You can help your parent reduce their financial burden by using the list of prescription resources in the reference section of the book (Chapter 8: Resource Guide). Help your parent find a program that offers the most benefit for the specific prescriptions.

For School Nurses

Wow, do you have a big job! You're responsible for the individual care plans of hundreds of kids, with a range of conditions and at varying stages of development. You may even cover multiple schools or only be with each group of kids 1 day a week.

Diabetes alone can present a huge challenge. Kids will be on different forms of insulin, with some using injections and others using insulin pumps. Some families may be very involved while others may take a more hands-off approach. Not to mention, you may be responsible for educating the teachers and support staff, too. You'll likely be managing these aspects of diabetes care in addition to helping kids with asthma, life-threatening food allergies, and a host of other conditions.

First we'd like to say thank you for reading this book and for being the amazing people that you are, by doing so much with so few resources. As a school nurse, you play a key role in supporting a child's successful transition from parent care to self-care. You are in the unique position of being a respected, neutral person who is in a position of authority. You have the ability to give instruction and teach without the emotional entanglement that often happens when parents try to teach their kids.

For parents of kids with diabetes, particularly type 1, leaving their children in the care of others is incredibly stressful. Parents are full of fear and anxiety, and these emotions can sometimes be directed at you. Thank you for recognizing this and for having grace and patience when dealing with anxious parents.

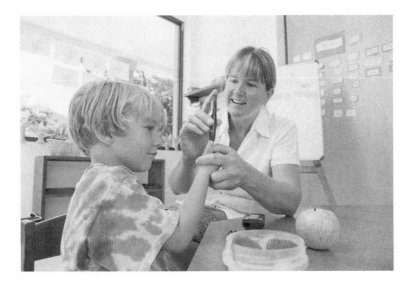

Having a clear and realistic plan for communication about blood glucose management between the school and parents can defuse frustration and tension. Depending on the age of the child, this communication may be daily, weekly, or only if blood glucose levels are outside a specified range. The key is to work together to define that plan and then use technology to keep the administrative burden to a minimum. Individual Education Plans (IEPs) and 504 plans are designed to capture and support the individual needs of students. When working with parents to develop a care plan, to reduce confusion and friction, be specific about addressing how you're going to communicate about supplies, changes in regular schedules/special events, substitute nurses or teachers, or protocols for high and low blood glucose levels.

This book covers many aspects of diabetes management that will help in your work with kids with diabetes (and parents), but here are four areas of particular importance:

1. The American Diabetes Association has wonderful resources for schools. Their Safe at School collection contains videos, handouts, and quick reference guides that can keep the *ADA Standards of Care, Safe at School,* and 504 plan guidelines at your fingertips. They also provide tools to use to facilitate

---

What Are IEPs and 504 Plans?

These plans are developed to ensure that a child who has a disability identified under the law and is attending an elementary or secondary educational institution receives accommodations that will ensure academic success and access to the learning environment.

education for support staff, other students, and families on the topic of diabetes.

2. Kids living with diabetes can still eat sugar and carbohydrates. Carbohydrates are the primary source of fuel for the brain and other organs and are necessary for healthy growth and development. Individuals will have different guidelines for meal plans, but the common goal is to strive to balance carbs, activity, and insulin to keep blood glucose levels in the target range as often as possible.

3. Kids who live with type 1 diabetes and wear an insulin pump are at greater risk of diabetic ketoacidosis (DKA). Insulin pumps only use fast-acting insulin, which leaves the body's system in about 3–4 hours. Site failures or disconnecting from an insulin pump for more than 60 minutes can cause ketones and, if left untreated, DKA can develop. DKA is a serious condition that requires immediate medical attention and can be life-threatening (see page 175 to learn more about DKA).

    Because technology changes so quickly, the best resource for information on insulin pumps and CGMs is the device manufacturer. The most common brands are:

    - Medtronic (pump and/or integrated Medtronic CGM)
    - OmniPod (pump)
    - Tandem (pump and/or integrated Dexcom CGM)
    - Dexcom (CGM)

    Each of these companies offers complimentary support materials for device users and their family and support team. Visit their website or call the toll-free number on the device for assistance.

4. A diagnosis of diabetes for a child puts significant stress on a family—sometimes more than they can effectively manage. If you see a family struggling, work with your school or district social worker or counselor to help the family connect with additional resources in the community.

KEY POINTS

➤ Diabetes doesn't define your loved one with diabetes, but it is a part of his or her everyday life.

➤ Having the physical ability to do something, like check blood glucose, is vastly different from having the maturity to do it.

➤ Planning and preparation are the secret weapons to get kids ready to safely participate in activities away from home.

➤ Remove emotion and set a calm, matter-of-fact tone around diabetes tasks.

➤ Provide help that is helpful. Talk with your loved one to understand what support he or she finds helpful.

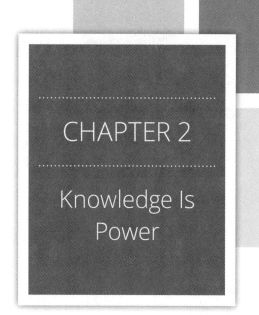

CHAPTER 2

Knowledge Is Power

During his presidential inauguration, Franklin D. Roosevelt uttered these famous words: "The only thing we have to fear is fear itself."

As much as we admire FDR and all he did for our country, we'd like to amend that statement slightly to include a little something about "the unknown."

Fear of the unknown can make us do some crazy things. Think about it. Much of the hatred in the world can be traced back to a lack of understanding and appreciation for different races and cultures. Many business people kick themselves for failing to invest in innovative products and ideas just because they were "out of the ordinary." And every day, we generate countless prejudices and fears toward people whose health conditions we don't quite understand.

Yes, the unknown *is* something to be feared. Before a lack of understanding of diabetes gets in the way of your ability to deal with it (and the people who have it) effectively, let's get to know it really, really well.

In this section, we will explain, in clear terms, exactly what diabetes is. We will reveal the true underlying causes of diabetes: who tends to get it, and why. We will explore the short-term and long-term effects of unmanaged diabetes. Along the way we will uncover many of the factors in everyday life that affect blood glucose levels so that you can see what it takes to manage diabetes properly.

Di-a-What? (Diabetes Defined)

Diabetes refers to the body's inability to properly regulate blood glucose levels. Most of the food we eat, especially carbohydrates, is digested and converted into a simple sugar called *glucose.* The glucose derived from our food enters the bloodstream and is carried to all parts of the body so that it can be burned for energy.

It is important to keep blood glucose levels within a certain range so that the body functions properly. If the blood glucose level is too low, the body's cells starve for energy. This is called *hypoglycemia* (hypo = low; glyc = sugar; emia = blood). If the blood glucose level is too high, blood vessels become clogged and damaged, and our whole body chemistry gets a bit out of whack. This is called *hyperglycemia* (hyper = high, and you know the rest).

Think of it this way: If you are making lemonade and put in too little sugar, the lemonade is going to taste sour. If you put in too much sugar, it will taste disgustingly sweet. Having just the right *concentration* of sugar is essential for making it taste just right. Having the right concentration of sugar (or glucose) in the bloodstream allows the body to function just right.

Insulin is very important to the whole process of blood glucose control. That's because glucose is a large molecule;

it can't get into most of the body's cells without a little help. Insulin provides that help. Insulin acts like a key that opens doors to the body's cells to allow those large glucose molecules to get inside. Get it? INsulin. INto cells.

FACTOID #1

Insulin's job is to take sugar (or glucose) out of the bloodstream and pack it into the body's cells to be burned for energy.

Insulin is made by the pancreas, an organ located just below the stomach. The pancreas constantly measures blood glucose levels and produces just enough insulin to keep the blood glucose within a normal range (approximately 60–100 mg/dL). As blood glucose levels go up, especially after meals, the pancreas makes more insulin. As blood

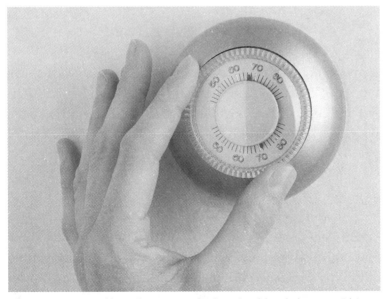

The pancreas acts like a thermostat for keeping blood glucose within a healthy range, using insulin to lower it and glucagon to raise it.

glucose levels drop, the pancreas makes less insulin. These changes occur between meals and when we are physically active. If blood glucose levels drop too much, the pancreas makes *glucagon*, a hormone that helps to raise blood glucose levels quickly.

The pancreas acts in a sense like the thermostat in your home. Let's say you set the thermostat for 70 degrees. When the temperature starts to rise, as often happens on a sunny day or during the summer, the thermostat turns the fan and air conditioner on until the temperature gets back down close to 70. When the temperature starts to drop, as occurs overnight or in the wintertime, the thermostat kicks the heat on until the temperature gets up to about 70. In regulating our body's blood glucose level, the pancreas is the thermostat. Insulin is the air conditioner, and glucagon is the heat. So what could possibly go wrong? Unfortunately, plenty.

What Type Are You?

Diabetes occurs when blood glucose levels rise well above normal. Diabetes can be caused by two completely different problems. Either not enough insulin is produced by the pancreas, or the insulin that is produced just doesn't work very well.

Type 1 Diabetes

When someone has **type 1 diabetes**, the pancreas stops making insulin entirely, or almost entirely (many people with type 1 diabetes still make a little bit of their own insulin, but it's not nearly enough to control blood glucose levels properly). The part of the pancreas that produces insulin is destroyed, accidentally, by the body's own immune system. That's why type 1 diabetes is called an *autoimmune* disease. The immune system is supposed to attack things that don't belong in our bodies, such as bacteria and viruses, and should recognize parts of our own body and leave them alone. But in some people, the immune system does a poor job of differentiating between the "good guys" (our body's own parts) and the "bad guys" (bacteria and viruses). While hunting for bad guys, the immune system may accidentally attack some good guys . . . sort of like firing bullets randomly into a big crowd of people when trying to catch an escaping bank robber. Because the pancreas is the only part of the body that can produce insulin, an autoimmune attack on the pancreas leaves the body without this essential hormone.

With no insulin available, most of the body's cells do not get the glucose they need to survive, even though there is a great deal of it floating around in the bloodstream. People with type 1 diabetes require insulin injections to both survive and manage blood glucose levels. Type 1 diabetes used to be called "juvenile diabetes" because it was often diagnosed during childhood. However, about half of all cases of type 1 diabetes are diagnosed during adulthood, so we now just call it type 1 diabetes.

Type 2 Diabetes

More than 90% of people with diabetes have **type 2 diabetes.** Type 2 diabetes is very different from type 1 diabetes in that there is no autoimmune attack, and the pancreas continues to produce insulin. In fact, the pancreas may actually produce *more* insulin than in a person who does not have diabetes. This will make more sense as we look at what is really behind the development of type 2 diabetes.

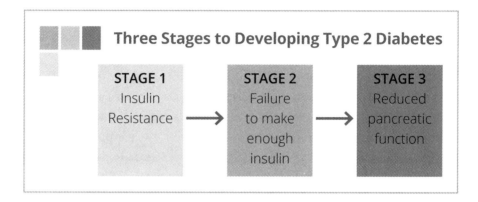

Three Stages to Developing Type 2 Diabetes

STAGE 1	STAGE 2	STAGE 3
Insulin Resistance	Failure to make enough insulin	Reduced pancreatic function

Stage 1: Le Résistance

To do its job of taking glucose out of the bloodstream and packing it into the body's cells, insulin attaches to "receptors" on the surface of our body's cells—similar to the way a key enters a lock to open a door. Once insulin attaches to the receptor, a series of chemical reactions take place, allowing the glucose molecules to enter the cell, just like turning a key causes a door to open.

For insulin to work, there have to be sufficient receptors on the cell surface, and the chemical reactions inside the cell have to occur properly. When there are problems with the receptors or the chemical reactions (like the key not fitting in the lock exactly right or the door being jammed), we enter a state of **insulin resistance.** When the body's cells are insulin resistant, insulin becomes less effective at lowering blood glucose.

What causes insulin resistance? Typically, it is a combination of genetics (our heredity) and lifestyle (the way we live our lives). Family history plays a major role. Having close relatives (parents, grandparents, aunts/uncles, siblings) with type 2 diabetes greatly increases your risk of becoming insulin resistant. Certain ethnic groups, including Native Americans, African Americans, Hispanic Americans, Asian Americans, and Pacific Islanders are also at a high risk. The aging process

POP QUIZ

Type 2 diabetes is:

A. Worse than type 1 diabetes.

B. The "not so bad" form of diabetes.

C. Preventable in some but not all people.

ANSWER: **C.** All forms of diabetes can cause serious health problems and create challenges to daily living. But unlike type 1 diabetes, which is not yet preventable, type 2 diabetes can, in many cases, be delayed or prevented through lifestyle changes.

plays a role as well. The older we get, the more insulin resistant we tend to become.

Women who have polycystic ovarian syndrome (PCOS) often become insulin resistant due to the overproduction of hormones that oppose insulin's action. Likewise, growth and hormones produced during pregnancy oppose insulin's action and cause insulin resistance. Gestational diabetes is a form of diabetes that usually goes away at the end of pregnancy. However, women who have had gestational diabetes during pregnancy are at an increased risk for developing type 2 diabetes later in life.

Stressful circumstances, such as illnesses, injuries, surgical procedures, or daily emotional turmoil, can cause insulin resistance. A number of medications can also produce insulin resistance: most notably anti-inflammatory "steroid" drugs, such as cortisone and prednisone, and a number of treatments for asthma.

A lack of physical activity can be a major source of insulin resistance. The muscles are one of the prime consumers of sugar for energy. When one's daily activity involves little more than getting up to find the remote control or car keys, muscles start to lose their sensitivity to insulin. Even in people who are usually very active, a couple of days without much activity will result in a decrease in insulin sensitivity.

Last but certainly not least, insulin resistance increases with body size. But let's get the terminology straight. We're not talking about being big and muscular. We're talking about having too much body fat, particularly around the middle. There is a direct link between the amount of body fat and the degree of insulin resistance.

FACTOID #2

More body fat = more insulin resistance.

More than 50 million Americans are considered to be obese (excessively fat). Obese individuals are more likely to develop diabetes than people who maintain a healthy body weight. And the problem is not restricted to adults. More than ever before, overweight children and teenagers are developing insulin resistance and type 2 diabetes.

Stage 2: The Production Shortfall

Insulin resistance affects at least 90 million Americans. Why, then, do only some people with insulin resistance develop type 2 diabetes? Sure, the number of people with type 2 diabetes is growing at a pretty fast pace (5% per year), but only about 20 million Americans are currently diagnosed with type 2 diabetes. Here's why.

When insulin resistance occurs, the pancreas usually produces enough extra insulin to keep blood glucose levels in a normal range, even though the insulin is not working as well as it should. This is called **prediabetes**.

But not everyone's pancreas has this capacity. Each person's pancreas can only crank up insulin production so much. Once the degree of insulin resistance is too much for the pancreas to overcome, blood glucose levels rise above normal. In other words, you must have both insulin resistance *and* a limit to the pancreas's ability to secrete extra insulin for type 2 diabetes to develop.

FACTOID #3

The combination of insulin resistance and a limited-capacity pancreas is what leads to type 2 diabetes.

To understand this concept better, recall our thermostat example. Imagine that you are an air conditioner trying to keep the house cool on a hot, humid summer day. If you're one of those high-powered central air conditioning units that can crank out tons of cold air, you'll have no problem overcoming the heat and keeping the house cool. But if you're a rusty old window unit, you're probably not going to be able to blow enough cold air to keep the entire house comfortable.

In this example, the heat and humidity represent insulin resistance, and the air conditioner is the pancreas. An efficient system can overcome the challenge, but a less efficient system will be unable to meet the challenge. When a sluggish pancreas meets major insulin resistance, the result is type 2 diabetes.

At this early phase of type 2 diabetes, blood glucose control can often be maintained through exercise and a healthy diet. Physical activity helps make the body's cells more sensitive to insulin. Consuming fewer carbohydrates (and the right *kind* of carbs) helps to limit the amount of glucose entering the bloodstream. And the combination of exercise and reduced calorie intake produces weight loss, which also improves insulin sensitivity. Sometimes, an oral medication can be used at this early phase of diabetes to supplement one's lifestyle efforts. But chances are, it won't do the job for long.

Stage 3: The Snowball Effect

Type 2 diabetes is a progressive illness. That is *not* a good thing. It grows worse and becomes harder to control over time. After having diabetes for a number of years, even with your best efforts, insulin resistance tends to grow worse, and the pancreas struggles to keep up with the huge demand for insulin. Then a new problem sets in. Just like our air conditioner that is forced to run full-blast every minute of every day, the pancreas starts to wear down. (If you were forced to work day after day without any breaks and no end in sight, you would wear down, too!)

The wearing-down of the pancreas is caused by two things: being overworked and a condition called *glucose toxicity*. The overworked part, we can all understand. Force that poor little pancreas into relentless slave labor, and eventually it will wear out. Glucose toxicity is a bit more complex.

Glucose is a good thing in the right amounts. But too much of a good thing can be harmful. High blood glucose can actually damage the pancreas, further reducing its ability to produce insulin. So over time, as a result of the constant battle against insulin resistance and high blood glucose, the pancreas starts to make less and less insulin.

This is why treating type 2 diabetes usually requires additional and more complex treatments over time. Additional medications may be required (in addition to a healthy lifestyle). In fact, 40% of people with type 2 diabetes take insulin to help control their blood glucose levels, sometimes several times each day or by using an insulin pump. Does this mean they now have type 1 diabetes? No, it does not. The type of diabetes you have is defined by what *caused* it, not how it is treated. Type 1 diabetes occurs when the body's immune system destroys the part of the pancreas that makes insulin. Type 2 diabetes is caused by insulin resistance, combined with insufficient insulin production, followed by a gradual breakdown of the pancreas.

Why Bother?

You might be reading this and thinking to yourself, "So what? What's the big deal if blood glucose levels are higher than normal?" Unfortunately, a lot of things go wrong when blood glucose levels are too high. If you've ever had cotton candy or spilled something sweet like juice or regular soda, you know how sticky sugar can be. In the bloodstream, excess sugar (glucose) makes the blood harder for the heart to pump. High glucose levels cause the unhealthy LDL fats to stick to the walls of blood vessels, making them stiffer, less elastic, and narrower. Glucose also sticks to cells and proteins in the bloodstream, causing them to function abnormally. When the body's vital organs are exposed to too much glucose, they

POP QUIZ

A person with type 2 diabetes who needs to take insulin:

A. Has turned into a person with type 1 diabetes.

B. Must give up everything they enjoy.

C. Still has type 2 diabetes.

ANSWER: C. Remember, the type of diabetes you have is determined by what caused it, not how you treat it. And taking insulin should definitely not force you to avoid the things you enjoy!

may become damaged or susceptible to infection (viruses and bacteria just *love* all that glucose!).

As a result, poorly controlled diabetes contributes to a number of major long-term health problems:

➤ Heart disease

➤ Stroke

➤ Poor circulation in the feet and legs

➤ Kidney disease

➤ Impaired vision and blindness

➤ Nerve problems (lack of sensation or constant pain)

➤ Sexual dysfunction

➤ Impaired digestion

➤ Loss of balance

➤ Gum disease

➤ Depression

➤ Memory problems

➤ "Frozen" joints

And that's not all. In the short term, the quality of one's daily life can be influenced by poorly controlled diabetes. The ability to feel good and perform well may be affected. High blood glucose levels can have a negative impact on the following:

➤ Energy levels

➤ Sleep patterns

➤ Strength and stamina

➤ Appetite control

➤ Mental sharpness

➤ Moods

➤ Ability to fight illness/infection

So clearly, there are many good reasons to do what is necessary to manage blood glucose levels. Almost every aspect of our physical, intellectual, and emotional well-being depends on it.

....

The Balancing Act

When it comes right down to it, managing blood glucose levels is like performing a balancing act. Our job is to balance the factors that raise blood glucose against the factors that lower it, with a goal of keeping the blood glucose within a healthy

Things that raise blood glucose: food, stress, illness, insulin resistance

Things that lower blood glucose: insulin, diabetes medications, physical activity

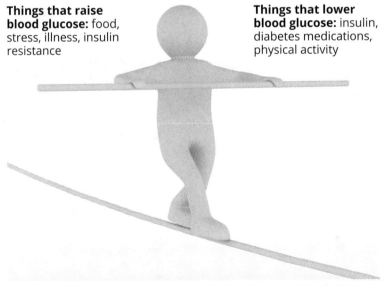

Managing diabetes involves balancing factors that raise blood glucose against the factors that lower blood glucose.

range (as recommended by your physician) as often as possible. As you'll learn later in this book, *perfect* blood glucose control is not necessary and indeed not possible. *Reasonable* control, in which blood glucose levels are in-range the majority of the time, is the usual goal.

SECRET STRATEGY #1

Remember, perfection isn't necessary!

If it helps, consider that an all-star baseball player only gets a hit 3 out of 10 times at-bat. A Pro Bowl quarterback only completes about 60% of his passes. And the best basketball players struggle to make 50% of their shots. Talk with your health care team about how often you should expect your blood glucose levels to be in-range. (Hint: it isn't 100%!)

Let's start out by looking at some of the major factors that affect your blood glucose.

Factors That Raise and Lower Blood Glucose Levels

Raise Blood Glucose	Lower Blood Glucose
⇧ Food (especially carbs)	⇩ Physical activity
⇧ The liver (via stress hormones)	⇩ Insulin
	⇩ Other diabetes medications

QUOTE OF THE CENTURY

"Three horses draw the diabetic chariot and their names are diet, exercise, and insulin."

– Elliot P. Joslin, MD, the first doctor in the U.S. to specialize in diabetes

Factor 1: Food

Whoever said that there is no such thing as a free lunch really knew what they were talking about. It seems like almost everything we eat or drink can cause blood glucose levels to rise.

The three major nutrients found in food are protein, fat, and carbohydrate. Carbohydrates are the nutrients that have the greatest effect on blood glucose levels. Carbohydrates (or "carbs") include simple sugars like glucose, sucrose (table sugar), fructose (fruit sugar), and lactose (milk sugar), as well as complex carbohydrates, better known as "starches." Most starches are composed of many glucose molecules linked together. Think of simple sugars as individual railroad cars and starch as a whole bunch of cars connected to make a train.

Carbohydrates

Now here is a statement you'll want to read several times. From the standpoint of blood glucose management, **it doesn't matter if the carbohydrates you eat are in the form of sugars or starches. Both will raise blood glucose by the same amount.** A cup of rice containing 45 grams of complex carbohydrate (starch) will raise blood glucose just as much as a can of regular (non-diet) soda that contains 45 grams of simple carbohydrate (sugar). And in this case, both will do it pretty fast. The fact is, in most cases, the amount of carbohydrate is more important than the type.

In addition to the items listed above, non-starchy vegetables have a small amount of carbohydrate. "Protein" foods such as meats, cheeses, and eggs have little to no carbohydrate.

Also, be aware that some "sugar-free" products contain carbohydrates that can raise blood glucose. Advertising people will do just about anything to get you to buy their products—even if it means bending the truth a little. "Sugar-free" can be put on a food label if the food does not contain

Foods Rich in Carbohydrates

Foods Rich in Sugar (simple carbohydrates)	Foods Rich in Starch (complex carbohydrates)
Fruit	Potatoes
Fruit juice	Rice
Raisins/dried fruit	Noodles/pasta
Regular soda	Cereal
Sports drinks	Oatmeal
Candy	Bread
Chocolate	Crackers
Cookies	Bagels
Cake	Pizza
Pies and pastries	Tortillas
Muffins	Pancakes
Milk	Waffles
Ice cream	Beans
Yogurt	Peas
Sport drinks	Corn
Table sugar	Pretzels
Honey	Chips
Syrup	Popcorn
Jelly	Matzoh

sucrose (table sugar). However, a sugar-free food can contain complex carbohydrates, fructose (fruit sugar), and a variety of "sugar substitutes" such as sorbitol, xylitol, mannitol, lactitol, isomalt, and maltodextrin, all of which raise blood glucose levels.

FACTOID #4

A bagel-shop bagel will raise blood glucose about as much as two plain donuts.

There are only a few artificial sweeteners that have no significant effect on blood glucose levels. These include saccharin, acesulfame K, sucralose, and aspartame. But once again, be careful. Products that contain these artificial sweeteners may also contain other sugar substitutes or carbohydrates that will raise your blood glucose level. The bottom line: Always read the nutrition label and look for the total carbohydrate (as well as the serving size). Even though carbohydrates raise blood glucose, they should not be viewed as "the enemy." Remember, blood glucose control is about balance. We simply need to balance what raises the blood glucose (such as carbs) against something that lowers it (such as insulin, medication, or physical activity).

It is worth noting that not all carbs are created equal. Some carbs, such as those found in candy and regular soda, don't have the nutritional value of carbs found in foods like fruit and whole-grain breads. Also, certain carbs raise blood glucose levels faster than others. This is important, because the slower a food raises blood glucose, the easier it is to keep blood glucose levels from spiking too high after eating.

Glycemic index (GI) is a term used to measure the *rate* at which carbohydrates convert into blood glucose. While virtually all carbohydrates convert into blood glucose eventually, some convert much faster than others. Most starchy foods (bread, rice, cereal, potatoes) have a relatively high GI; they digest easily and convert into blood glucose quickly. Exceptions include starches found in pasta and legumes. Foods that have dextrose in them tend to have a very high GI. Fructose (fruit sugar) and lactose (milk sugar) are slower to convert into blood glucose than most starches. Table sugar (sucrose) has a moderate GI, as do most mixed meals. Vegetables (other than potatoes) tend to have low GI values. Foods that contain fiber or large amounts of fat tend to have lower GI values than foods that do not. Understanding how the body responds to different types of carbs plays a key role in knowing which ones to use in which situation. Knowledge is power! If you are trying to quickly raise your blood glucose, reach for something that has a very high GI. If you are looking for sustained energy/blood glucose, choose something that has a lower GI.

Protein

Protein, which is found in meats, dairy products, eggs, nuts, and soy, has a minimal effect on blood glucose, but there are a few exceptions. When very little carbohydrate is consumed, some dietary protein is converted to glucose by the liver. For example, if you wake up to a breakfast of nothing but eggs and sausage, you may see a noticeable blood glucose rise a few hours later. However, when carbohydrate is present in a meal or snack, protein has little to no effect on blood glucose, unless there is a *very* large amount of protein in the meal (more than 50–60 grams of protein). This is equivalent to more than 9 ounces of meat or nine eggs. When consuming large amounts of protein, some of the protein will raise the blood glucose level.

Fat

Dietary fat's immediate impact on blood glucose is usually insignificant. However, consumption of large amounts of fat can cause two distinct effects. First, it may slow the digestion of the carbohydrates that were consumed along with the fat. And second, large amounts of dietary fat, particularly saturated fat, can produce short-term insulin resistance, which may raise the blood glucose level over a period of many hours.

 FACTOID #5

Large amounts of fat in a meal or snack may slow the digestion of carbohydrate and produce a secondary blood glucose rise after the carbohydrates have finished digesting.

Factor 2: Stress Hormones

Last weekend, one of our patients decided to stay up late and watch a scary movie. It was one of those super-gross zombie movies where the zombies eat the flesh of unsuspecting vacationers. After the final gut-wrenching, heart-pumping scene, our patient decided to check his blood glucose. It had *risen* about 200 mg/dL (11 mmol/L) during the movie. With blood that sweet, he may have been the grand prize for any zombies who might be lurking in the neighborhood! The big mystery was, if he didn't eat during the movie (he was probably too nauseated), where did the sugar come from?

Enter the liver. Everyone's liver serves as a storehouse for glucose, keeping it in a concentrated form called *glycogen*. The liver breaks down small amounts of glycogen all the time, releasing glucose into the bloodstream to nourish the brain, nerves, heart, and other "always active" organs.

The liver's release of glucose is affected by certain hormones. Of all the hormones in the body, only insulin causes the liver to take sugar out of the bloodstream and store it. All the other hormones—including stress hormones, sex hormones, growth hormones, and glucagon—cause the liver to secrete glucose back into the bloodstream.

Cortisol and growth hormone are produced in a 24-hour cycle and are responsible for the blood glucose rise that we sometimes see during the night or in the early morning (this is referred to as a "dawn effect"). The other "stress" hormones, particularly epinephrine (adrenaline), are produced when our body needs a rapid influx of sugar for energy purposes. The glucose rise our patient experienced during the scary movie was no doubt caused by stress hormones.

Emotional stress (fear, anxiety, anger, excitement, tension) and physiological stress (illness, pain, infection, injury) cause the body to produce stress hormones. For people without diabetes, the stress-induced blood glucose rise is followed by an increase in insulin secretion, so the blood glucose rise is modest and temporary. For people with diabetes, however, stress can cause a significant and prolonged increase in the blood glucose level.

Factor 3: Physical Activity

Physical activity is a potent tool for lowering blood glucose. It does this by burning glucose and improving the way insulin works. Remember . . . insulin is like a key that opens "doors" to your body's cells, allowing sugar to enter and be burned for energy. When you've been lying around like a sloth, your muscle cells don't need much energy, so they only have a few doors available to open. Now, imagine that you decide to do your own gardening and yardwork—you, yourself, who has no real outdoor skills whatsoever. All of a sudden, your muscle cells need lots more energy. The few doors that exist on your muscle cells don't allow the sugar to get inside fast enough. The solution, as you might have guessed, is for your body's cells to make more doors and "grease the hinges." And that's just what happens.

Suddenly, those insulin keys find it much easier to open doors and shuttle glucose out of the bloodstream and into

---

POP QUIZ

Stress tends to make blood glucose levels:

A. Go up

B. Go down

C. I'm too stressed out to care

ANSWER: **A.** Stress hormones cause the liver to secrete glucose into the bloodstream, resulting in a blood glucose rise.

your cells, giving you the energy to clean up the huge mess in the yard. Unfortunately, nothing lasts forever. The extra "doors" built by the body's cells are only temporary. After being sedentary for a couple of days, many of the doors are taken away and you return to the way things were before your activity level increased. In fact, extended periods of inactivity can reduce your sensitivity to insulin, resulting in a state of insulin resistance. This, as we discussed, is a major characteristic of type 2 diabetes. But it can happen to people with type 1 diabetes as well.

As for burning glucose, the body burns lots and lots of it during exercise. Depending on your body size and the nature of your physical activity, you might burn upwards of 100 grams of glucose per hour!

You've probably heard that blood glucose can go *up* during exercise. And it's true—it can. But it is not the physical activity that causes it. Physical activity *always* burns sugar and improves insulin sensitivity. Something else is going on at the same time: a "stress response." This response can take place during competitive activities, very-high-intensity/short-duration exercises, judged performances, and sports that involve quick bursts of movement. If the blood glucose rise from the stress response is greater than the glucose burned by working muscles, the net result can be a rise in the blood glucose level.

Factor 4: Insulin

Insulin lowers blood glucose. Plain and simple. Insulin produced by the pancreas works very quickly, within just a few seconds after it is produced, and finishes working within a few minutes. Insulin taken by injection varies in terms of its onset (start) of action, its peak action time (when it lowers blood glucose the fastest), and its duration (when it completely finishes working). But there is no injected insulin that works nearly as quickly as insulin produced by the body. Inhaled insulin's speed of action falls somewhere between that of injected insulin and the body's natural insulin.

A summary of insulin types is given below. Be aware that the precise action times can vary from person to person.

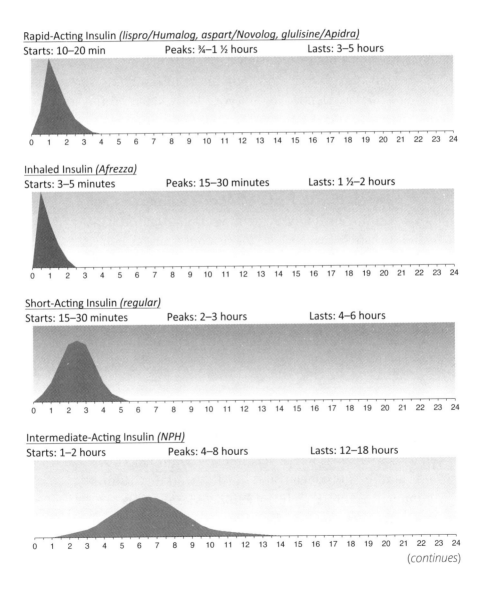

Rapid-Acting Insulin *(lispro/Humalog, aspart/Novolog, glulisine/Apidra)*
Starts: 10–20 min   Peaks: ¾–1 ½ hours   Lasts: 3–5 hours

Inhaled Insulin *(Afrezza)*
Starts: 3–5 minutes   Peaks: 15–30 minutes   Lasts: 1 ½–2 hours

Short-Acting Insulin *(regular)*
Starts: 15–30 minutes   Peaks: 2–3 hours   Lasts: 4–6 hours

Intermediate-Acting Insulin *(NPH)*
Starts: 1–2 hours   Peaks: 4–8 hours   Lasts: 12–18 hours

(continues)

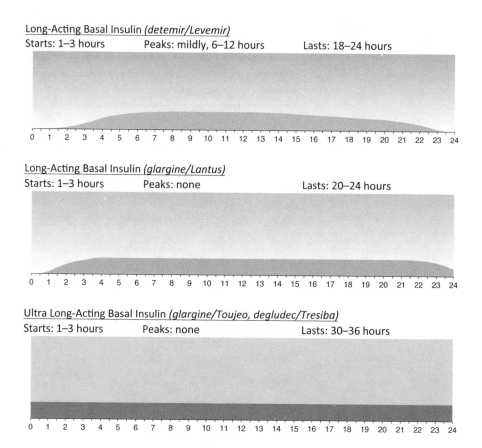

Long-Acting Basal Insulin *(detemir/Levemir)*
Starts: 1–3 hours   Peaks: mildly, 6–12 hours   Lasts: 18–24 hours

Long-Acting Basal Insulin *(glargine/Lantus)*
Starts: 1–3 hours   Peaks: none   Lasts: 20–24 hours

Ultra Long-Acting Basal Insulin *(glargine/Toujeo, degludec/Tresiba)*
Starts: 1–3 hours   Peaks: none   Lasts: 30–36 hours

Premixed insulins, such as 75/25, 70/30, and 50/50, contain a combination of NPH (intermediate-acting insulin) and either regular or rapid-acting insulin. For example, Humalog Mix 75/25 contains 75% NPH and 25% Humalog. Novolin 70/30 contains 70% NPH and 30% regular insulin.

Factor 5: "Other" Diabetes Medications

Diabetes medications come in two forms: pills and injectables. Obviously, one of the injectables is insulin. But there are other injectables that are used to treat diabetes. See pages 66–67 for a summary of the currently available medications.

Oral Medications (Pills)

Drug Class	Examples (brand names in parentheses)	How They Work
Biguanides	metformin (Glucophage) metformin XR (Glumetza, Fortamet) metformin liquid (Riomet)	Keeps the liver from producing too much glucose
Sulfonylureas	chlorpropamide (Diabinese) glyburide (Diabeta, glynase, Micronase) glipizide (Glucotrol, Glucotrol XL) glimepiride (Amaryl) tolazamide tolbutamide	Stimulates the pancreas to make more insulin for 12–24 hours
Meglitinides	repaglinide (Prandin) nateglinide (Starlix)	Stimulates the pancreas to make more insulin for 2–4 hours
Thiazoladinediones	pioglitazone (Actos) rosiglitazone (Avandia)	Increases muscle and fat cells' sensitivity to insulin
α-Glucosidase inhibitors	acarbose (Precose) miglitol (Glyset)	Inhibits the digestion of carbohydrates
DPP-4 (dipeptidyl peptidase-4) inhibitors	sitagliptin (Januvia) saxagliptin (Onglyza) linagliptin (Tradjenta) alogliptin (Nesina)	Slows digestion, blunts appetite, stimulates the pancreas, blocks glucagon production
SGLT-2 (sodium–glucose cotransporter-2) inhibitors	canagliflozin (Invokanna) empagliflozin (Jardiance) dapagliflozin (Farxiga)	Causes the kidneys to excrete glucose in the urine

(There are also pills that include combinations of two different oral medications listed above.)

Non-Insulin Injectables

Drug Class	Examples (brand names in parentheses)	How They Work
Amylin mimetics	pramlintide (Symlin)	Slows digestion, blunts appetite, blocks glucagon production
GLP-1 (glucagon-like peptide 1)	exenatide (Bydureon, Byetta) liraglutide (Victoza) lixisenatide (Lyxumia) dulaglitide (Trulicity)	Slows digestion, blunts appetite, stimulates the pancreas, blocks glucagon production

All diabetes medications have their share of benefits and potential drawbacks. If you're interested in learning more about a particular class of medications, talk to your physician.

Little Things That Affect Your Glucose Levels

There are countless variables that can affect blood glucose levels—some raising it, some lowering it, and some not always having a consistent pattern. Here's a partial list of things that can affect blood glucose levels.

More Things That Affect Blood Glucose Levels

Tend to Raise Blood Glucose	Tend to Lower Blood Glucose
Growth	Alcohol
Menstrual hormones	Heat/humidity
Later stages of pregnancy	Heavy brain work
Rebounds from hypoglycemia	Previous intense exercise
Gradual loss of β-cell function (type 2 diabetes)	New/unusual surroundings
Exiting the "honeymoon" period (type 1 diabetes)	Socializing
Depression	Stimulating environments (multiple areas of the brain and senses are being used at once)
Weight gain	Early stages of pregnancy

(continues)

More Things That Affect Blood Glucose Levels (*Continued*)

Tend to Raise Blood Glucose	Tend to Lower Blood Glucose
Excessive sleeping	β-Blockers
Caffeine	MAO (monoamine oxidase) inhibitors
Steroid medications	Nicotine patches
Diuretics	Ritalin
Estrogen	Stress reduction
Niacin	Reducing symptoms of depression

What About Hypoglycemia?

We've reviewed the factors involved in the "balancing act." Raise or lower things on one side of the scale and you need to match it with an increase or decrease on the other side. When an imbalance takes place, the result is either high or low blood glucose. We've discussed the causes and effects of high blood glucose in detail already. Now, let's take a brief look at the lows.

Low blood glucose, commonly known as *hypoglycemia*, occurs when the body's cells are deprived of enough glucose to function properly. Symptoms including shaking, sweating, rapid heartbeat, intense hunger, and a pale complexion. These symptoms usually occur when blood glucose levels fall below 70 mg/dL, but symptoms can appear at slightly higher glucose levels, especially in people whose blood glucose levels have been running high for quite some time. Symptoms of hypoglycemia may also appear when your blood glucose level drops very quickly from a high level toward normal.

Some parts of the body, such as the brain and nervous system, highly depend on glucose as a source of fuel. So when a drop in blood glucose occurs, the brain sends signals to the adrenal gland, which produces hormones that are supposed to help bring the blood glucose back up. Those same hormones also cause the symptoms described above. These signals should serve as a warning to the victim that his or her blood glucose is dropping, and food (rapid-acting carbohydrates) must be eaten right away. If food is not eaten, the blood glucose can continue to drop, resulting in confusion, mood changes, odd behavior, seizure, loss of consciousness, and, in extreme cases, even death. Hypoglycemia rarely occurs in people who are *not* taking insulin or one of the oral medications that cause the pancreas to secrete extra insulin (sulfonylureas and meglitinides). We'll discuss hypoglycemia in greater detail later on (see Chapter 7).

Self-Monitoring

An essential aspect of diabetes management is self-monitoring of blood glucose levels. Monitoring allows us to evaluate the effectiveness of the overall diabetes program as well as make necessary adjustments on a day-to-day basis.

There are a number of options for monitoring blood glucose. **Blood glucose meters** require the user to prick a finger

POP QUIZ

If you don't take insulin or a medication that stimulates the pancreas to make more insulin:

A. It is very unlikely that you will experience low blood glucose.

B. It is OK to let your blood glucose run a little above normal.

C. Your diabetes is not all that serious.

ANSWER: **A.** Unless you take insulin or a medication that can cause the pancreas to overproduce insulin, there is really no reason for low blood glucose to occur.

for a small blood sample. Some meters allow the user to obtain a very tiny blood sample from a less sensitive area such as the forearm. Meters provide immediate, point-in-time blood glucose measurements. **Continuous glucose monitors** use a sensor placed just below the skin to transmit readings wirelessly to a handheld receiver that displays ongoing readings. The receiver can also alert the user of pending highs and lows. And a lab test called an **A1C** (hemoglobin A1c) provides a 2- to 3-month "average" blood glucose based on the proportion of red blood cells that have glucose attached.

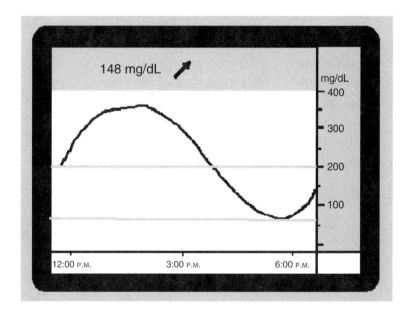

FACTOID #6

In ancient Egypt, the "physician" would detect diabetes by tasting the urine of afflicted individuals, since sugar passes into the urine when the blood glucose is elevated. No wonder there was a shortage of good physicians!

The frequency and nature of self-monitoring is highly individualized, based on one's goals, treatment plan, and potential risks. We'll discuss more about monitoring, and what to do with the information, later on.

KEY POINTS

➤ Diabetes comes in two forms: type 1 diabetes, caused by an autoimmune mishap, and type 2 diabetes, caused by insulin resistance and insufficient insulin production by the pancreas.

➤ Managing diabetes involves balancing the factors that raise blood glucose (food, stress) against the factors that lower it (physical activity, insulin, and other diabetes medications).

➤ Elevated blood glucose can cause many health problems in the long term and affects quality of life in the short term.

➤ People who take insulin or pancreas-stimulating medications are at risk for low blood glucose, which can be dangerous in the short term.

CHAPTER 3

The Art, Science, and Emotion of Diabetes Management

Diagnosis and Grief

Whether it's you or your loved one, a diagnosis of diabetes is a big blow that most people weren't expecting. When we talk about grief, many people think of it being related solely to the death of a loved one. While this is true, people also experience grief whenever there's a loss—of any kind.

Diabetes can represent the loss of a way of life that you once had, the loss of independence and freedom, the loss of what you thought childhood would or should look like, or the loss of how you viewed your health or the health of your loved one. With the potential for all of these feelings of loss, when you or someone you love is diagnosed with diabetes, there is a grieving process that you both go through.

Grief experts have identified seven stages of grieving. Knowing these phases will help you and your loved one understand some of your feelings related to the diagnosis and give a little bit of insight into what happens during the grieving process. But even with an understanding of the grief stages, it's important to realize that grief isn't linear, and different people will move through the stages at their own pace, possibly skipping stages or revisiting earlier ones.

The nonlinear part is important to understand because even though someone has moved past a certain stage, life events or triggers can send the person back to an earlier grief stage. Knowing this can help you understand why someone appears to be so angry about diabetes when, just a few months ago, it seemed like he or she had adjusted to the diagnosis. Keeping in mind the individual pace of progress through the grief stages can prevent you from trying to get your loved one to operate in one stage when he or she is still in an earlier stage.

The Seven Stages of Grief

1. Shock and denial

You will probably react to learning of the loss with numbed disbelief. You may deny the reality of the loss at some level to avoid the pain. Shock provides emotional protection from being overwhelmed all at once. This may last for weeks.

2. Pain and guilt

As the shock wears off, it is replaced with the suffering of pain. Although uncomfortable, it is important that you experience the pain fully, and not hide it, avoid it, or escape from it with alcohol or drugs. You may have guilty feelings or remorse for choices you did or didn't make. Life feels chaotic and scary during this phase.

3. Anger and bargaining

Frustration gives way to anger, and you may lash out and lay unwarranted blame for the diagnosis. This is a time for the release of bottled up emotion. You may rail against fate, questioning, "Why me?" You may also try to bargain in vain with the powers that be for a way out of your despair.

4. Depression, reflection, and loneliness

Just when your friends may think you should be getting on with your life, a long period of sad reflection will likely overtake you. This is a normal stage of grief, so do not be "talked out of it" by well-meaning outsiders. Encouragement from others is not helpful to you during this stage of grieving. During this time, you finally realize the true magnitude of your loss, and it depresses you. You may isolate yourself on purpose, reflect on things you did before your loss, and focus on memories of the past. You may sense feelings of emptiness or despair.

5. The upward turn

As you start to adjust to your new normal, your life becomes a little calmer and more organized. Your physical symptoms lessen, and your "depression" begins to lift slightly.

6. Reconstruction

As you become more functional, your mind starts working again, and you will find yourself seeking realistic solutions to problems posed by your new reality.

7. Acceptance and hope

During this last stage, you learn to accept and deal with the reality of your situation. Acceptance does not necessarily mean instant happiness. Life will never be exactly the same as before diagnosis, but you will find a way forward.

What's Your Diabetes Emotional Health?

Right from the start, emotional health plays an important role in life with diabetes. Chapter 2 mentioned A1C, what it means, and the role it plays in tracking how well a diabetes management plan is working for someone. Much of the focus around achieving and maintaining a target A1C is dedicated to the physiological (physical) parts of diabetes management.

Careful monitoring and adjustments are made to establish the correct combination of medication, food, and exercise that supports our body's ability to maintain steady(ish) blood glucose levels. While diabetes management does have a good measure of art to it, which we'll discuss as well, rest assured, there are some aspects of the equation that are proven to hold true for everybody.

For example, taking insulin reduces blood glucose levels. Eating foods containing carbohydrates raises blood glucose levels. This is part of the *science* of diabetes management. The *art* comes in the form of things like timing and amounts of insulin; factoring in things like excitement, illness, activity, and weather; and choreographing all of these moving pieces into a diabetes dance without falling off of the stage. Now that's art!

Most health care providers agree that effective diabetes management is both an art and a science. They will give you the basic facts and tools and then leave it to the person with diabetes to figure out the art.

As a mother of a child with diabetes, Diane wanted the recipe for perfect diabetes management. She wanted to do everything possible to make sure that her son's blood glucose levels stayed as close to "normal" as possible. It didn't matter how much effort it would take. She was willing to learn and do what was needed, recognizing that it would take modifying daily schedules and making significant lifestyle changes. The goal was to find the formula that would allow her son to live his life the way he would have without diabetes and to remain the same healthy kid he was before diabetes.

After a crusade to gather as much information and insight as possible about what the magic formula looked like, what most of the information available suggested was something like this:

Medication + Education + Technology and Tools
= Perfect Diabetes Control

Or does it? If there *is* a formula for achieving on-target blood glucose levels and A1C values, why do so many people living with diabetes still have levels that are well outside the target range and struggle to keep up with diabetes management tasks? This question has been the source of much debate and analysis and has led to a culture with a great deal of blame being placed on the person with diabetes.

Why won't they do what they are supposed to do?
Why do they eat that when they know what it will
do to their blood glucose? Why won't they take their
medications? They <u>know</u> they need to exercise
and lose weight, but they just won't.

This line of thinking drives health care professionals and family members to search for ways to get people with diabetes to do what they are *supposed* to do. For us, we didn't have to look further than our own situations to know that this formula is missing some key ingredients. To get this recipe to work, we needed to figure these ingredients out!

As part of our exploration into the missing ingredients in the *perfect diabetes management* recipe, we were struck by a group of people who are truly "diabetes heroes." These are our work associates who have lived with diabetes for literally decades, and in some cases for more than 50 years.

These people came into the world of diabetes at a time where there was no such thing as a glucose meter, let alone continuous glucose monitors. Syringes were glass with harpoon-like steel needles that required boiling and sharpening (literally). Insulin came in two forms: slow and slower. And very little was known about the interactions between different foods, exercise, emotions, and blood glucose levels. And yet, even with only the most primitive tools, this group of people managed to live full, active lives, complete with families, careers, travel, and a host of accomplishments. Essentially, they were able to thrive while living with diabetes.

The other thing we observed, is that we also work with an equal number of people who, by contrast, have access to all of the latest information and technologies to help "optimize" diabetes management. Yet they struggle to maintain diabetes management routines and blood glucose levels, and diabetes takes a significant toll on their physical and emotional health.

Most people want to feel well and be healthy. So what is it that allows some to thrive while others struggle, regardless of education, resources, age, or background? It turns out that the thing—the missing ingredient—is a collection of factors that have historically received little attention and support. The factors are the **emotional** aspects of living with diabetes.

SECRET STRATEGY #2

Ultimately, what separates those who thrive with diabetes from those who struggle is their approach to the emotional aspect of living with the disease.

It is important to understand the emotional and psychosocial factors that can and do affect diabetes management.

Let's break down "psychosocial" to get a better idea of the types of factors we're talking about: ***psycho*** = relating to the mind and ***social*** = relationships and interactions with family and society.

An important cornerstone of this book is the understanding that these factors that affect diabetes emotional health are a powerful part of the diabetes management equation and that it takes a healthy balance of effective glucose control and emotional wellness to thrive in the world of diabetes. There is a strong belief that when emotional health is taken care of, target A1C levels will follow. This book is about helping you and your loved one know how to support and care for both physical and emotional health.

So what are the emotional factors that affect diabetes, why do they matter, and what can we do to take care of our emotional health? This section will feature some of the common psychosocial issues associated with diabetes and provide steps you can take to protect against them and foster resilience for yourself and your loved one with diabetes.

....

Psychological Risks

Compared to individuals without diabetes, people with diabetes are at greater risk for depression, anxiety/panic attacks, and disordered eating. Additionally, people with diabetes often experience something known as diabetes distress, or "diabetes burnout." In fact, up to 48% of people with diabetes will experience high levels of diabetes distress in any 18-month period (Berg, EG. Sending out an SOS: Worried about your diabetes? You may have diabetes distress. *Diabetes Forecast,* June 2013: page 28).

Because you have a close relationship with someone who has diabetes, you may notice some warning signs or red flags well before he or she is even aware there is a problem. It's important that you share your concerns with the person and offer to help think through options for support—either from you or from a professional. We've identified specific things to look for and provide resources under each specific category.

There are many reasons that people don't feel comfortable having these types of difficult conversations, but having them can make a real difference for the person who is struggling. We later provide some conversation starters to help open the door to a constructive talk about your concerns.

While people with diabetes do have unique situations that can affect their emotional health, many strategies and tools discussed in this section are also useful to take care of yourself as well. This is particularly true when it comes to stress.

....

Stress: A Shared Reality

As we all know, stress isn't unique to people living with diabetes. We commonly make statements like, "I'm so stressed out" or "This stress is killing me." We recognize that we're experiencing stress, but how much do we know about how stress affects the body?

What Happens When You're Stressed?

During stressful situations, epinephrine (adrenaline), glucagon, growth hormone, and cortisol are all released to prepare the body for battle. Infections, illness, and emotional struggles are all seen as stressful situations by the body.

Chapter 2 covered in more depth what's going on physically during periods of stress, but here's a quick recap. The body's primary source of energy is glucose (sugar). So when under stress, the body ensures that there is enough sugar or energy available by lowering insulin levels and raising glucagon and epinephrine (adrenaline) levels. And finally the body dumps glucose stores from the liver. At the same time, growth hormone and cortisol levels rise, which causes body tissues (muscle and fat) to be less sensitive to insulin. As a result, more glucose is available in the bloodstream.

This "body magic" is just what you need when you're trying to outrun a grizzly bear that you encounter on a hike. But when commuting to work, or when a hectic schedule and daily life are provoking this same stress response, it's no longer a good thing and leads to health complications.

As a result of having all of these hormones firing off and having excess glucose in the blood, the stress response can cause irritability, food cravings, and difficulty sleeping. Prolonged periods of stress can also lead to weight gain (particularly unhealthy belly fat), insulin resistance, and other health issues. Stress can be a contributing factor in developing type 2 diabetes. We know from Chapter 2 that, for people with diabetes, stress raises blood glucose levels, increases insulin resistance, and makes blood glucose management more difficult.

Stress in modern life seems unavoidable. No one can fully insulate themselves from periods of illness, hectic schedules, and difficult life situations. To minimize the potential negative health effects of stress, it's important to find and adopt healthy ways to manage it.

Managing Stress

Stress management is an individual thing. One person's commune with nature is another person's battle with bugs and pollen. Take time to think about what reduces your stress and helps you relax. Regardless of which specific activities you find calming and enjoyable, here are some shared principles to use to reduce stress:

> ➤ **Movement:** Physical activity reduces stress, increases the release of endorphins (happy hormones), and boosts the immune system.

> ➤ **Meditation:** Meditation slows the pulse and heart rate, improves quality of breathing, and helps interrupt the escalation of the body's physical response to stress. Meditation can take many forms and doesn't have to be hours in a dark room in silence. *Headspace, MoodMeter,* and *Buddhify* are examples of apps that make it easy and fun to work meditation into daily routines. These apps can be downloaded to phones and computers.

> ➤ **Routines:** Having a routine helps automate aspects of our day and is a powerful way to reduce the stress that surrounds decisions, planning, and juggling tasks. Sticking to healthy sleep, exercise, and morning routines is a particularly effective way to manage and reduce stress.

There are many great books and resources that explain in more detail the importance of reducing stress and provide different ways to manage it. The message we're highlighting here is **don't minimize the importance of managing stress**. Finding ways to reduce stress will pay great dividends to physical, emotional, and relational health for both you and your loved one.

FACTOID #7

Diabetes distress refers to the unique, often hidden, emotional burdens and worries that patients experience when they are managing a severe chronic disease like diabetes. High levels of diabetes distress are common and distinct from clinical depression. Diabetes distress can also be experienced by partners and caregivers of people with diabetes because of their heavy involvement in diabetes management.

When experiencing diabetes distress, a person's levels of anxiety, worry, and fatigue can be particularly high, especially when it comes to diabetes care requirements and the topic of diabetes in general. Typically, people experiencing diabetes distress do not report feelings of anxiety and worry about other areas and aspects of their life. Rather, their distress is specific to diabetes. Below is a short screening tool that clinicians use to assess if a person might be in diabetes distress.

The 2-Item Diabetes Distress Screening Scale (DDS2)

Directions Living with diabetes can sometimes be tough. There may be many problems and hassles concerning diabetes and they can vary greatly in severity. Problems may range from minor hassles to major life difficulties. Listed below are 2 potential problem areas that people with diabetes may experience. Consider the degree to which each of the 2 items may have distressed or bothered you DURING THE PAST MONTH and circle the appropriate number.

Please note that we are asking you to indicate the degree to which each item may be bothering you in your life, NOT whether the item is merely true for you. If you feel that a particular item is not a bother or a problem for you, you would circle "1." If it is very bothersome to you, you might circle "6."

Feeling	Not a Problem		Moderate Problem		Serious Problem	
1. Feeling overwhelmed by the demands of living with diabetes.	1	2	3	4	5	6
2. Feeling that I am often failing with my diabetes regimen.	1	2	3	4	5	6

Reprinted with permission from the American Academy of Family Physicians: Appendix 2, Development of a Brief Diabetes Distress Screening Instrument, Page 246, written by Fisher, Lawrence, From *Annals of Family Medicine*, Published May/June 2008, Vol. 6, No. 3.

FACTOID #8

Diabetes burnout is the term given to the state of disillusion, frustration, and (sometimes) submission to the condition of diabetes and may be marked by a person's complete or partial disregard for blood glucose levels, eating habits, and/or medication requirements.

At some point, you may notice that your loved one with diabetes, who previously was on top of things, suddenly starts forgetting to check blood glucose or skips a few insulin doses and is otherwise acting like he or she doesn't have diabetes. This is a red flag that your loved one could be experiencing diabetes burnout.

Burnout can strike at any time. It does not matter if your loved one is a seasoned pro and has been managing diabetes for many years or he or she is new to the world of tracking, counting, adjusting, and managing blood glucose.

Your loved one understands the importance of maintaining consistent diabetes care routines. Therefore, reminding or nagging your loved one to maintain these routines frequently adds to the guilt he or she is feeling and reinforces the natural tendency to avoid unpleasant tasks. It's common for people with diabetes to at some point just decide that they can't or don't want to keep up with their diabetes care anymore. Pressure of work, raising children, managing the house, or getting through school can be physically and mentally draining. People need breaks from these routines and pressures to rejuvenate and reset. For these situations, we get respites through vacations, summer breaks, and babysitters. Unfortunately, there is no formal structure or term that allows a person with diabetes to take a break.

Diabetes is a 24/7/365 responsibility and almost everyone will experience some degree of diabetes burnout at some point. Having support from loved ones can be key to getting through those phases. One of the most important things you can do to support your loved one experiencing diabetes burnout is to resist the temptation to panic. Instead, *reframe the situation in your mind.*

SECRET STRATEGY #3

When a loved one is experiencing burnout, it is important that you not panic. Instead, take a step back and consider the context and factors that may be contributing to the situation.

What exactly is reframing?

Although it sounds like a complicated concept, reframing is actually something that we do all the time. A simple way to understand the concept of reframing is to consider how we use it to guide our thoughts and actions. We rely heavily on context to guide our opinion about a situation, remarks, or events. We can interpret the same event or situation completely differently when the context changes. For example, if you spot someone at the grocery store stealing an apple, your initial impression (the "panic" response) might be to assume that this person is a criminal and should be arrested to teach them a lesson. However, if you knew that this person had not eaten for days and had no money, you might offer to pay for the apple yourself.

Reframing has the power to change how we feel and perceive a situation or set of events. We can literally put a new frame around any situation and it will look and feel different. Reframing will help you support your loved ones with empathy and understanding rather than fear and anger. Simply knowing that it is common (and understandable) for people to become worn down by tasks that are repetitive and physically/emotionally draining, you will be in a position to offer more balanced help and support.

This is very different from looking at the situation with a frame or context of, "Why are they doing this? What's wrong with them? They should be taking care of their diabetes!" Worry and fear are real and understandable when someone you love lives with diabetes. But for the benefit of the emotional health of yourself and your loved one with diabetes, strive to take judgment out of diabetes management. When fear, anxiety, worry, and anger dominate our thinking, we fall into behaviors that create hurtful, counterproductive cycles. Staying "above the fray" is easier said than done (trust us, we know!), but the positive impact and results of making that switch are well worth the effort. Another benefit that comes from the flow of positive reinforcement is that when you react differently, they respond differently, breaking the gridlock that surrounds power struggles.

What does reframing really mean, and what does it look like? Let's reframe diabetes management not as a life-threatening medical condition, but as a job instead. Follow these scenarios below and see how reframing changes how you can view and react to a situation.

Boss Perspective:

"I can't believe you're taking a week off from work! Don't you know there are things around here that have to get done? We have customers, we have stockholders, and have you seen the numbers lately?! And you're going to take time off; are you kidding me? What are you thinking?!"

Most of us wouldn't expect this type of reaction at work if we took some time off. And if it were always like this, we would likely be looking for a new job. In a more positive employee/employer relationship (and one that is likely to last longer and get better results from the employee), the conversation might sound like this:

"Reframed" Boss Perspective:

"I can see that work has been pretty stressful lately, and you certainly deserve a break. Why don't you tell me what

you have on your plate so that we can make sure that it's covered while you're away."

Yes, diabetes is a medical condition, but diabetes management is a *job*. Diabetes happens to humans, not robots, and humans get run down and need to be able to recharge and, yes, "slack" off sometimes from their diabetes job. Being supported and able to take a "diabetes vacation" without feeling shame or guilt helps people recharge and come back from "vacation" ready to get back to routines and responsibilities.

The section below will give you some specific strategies to help your loved one through burnout. But as a word of caution, the person with diabetes must be ready to take these steps, and pushing him or her will likely make the situation worse. But regardless of your loved one's state of mind, you always have control over *your* actions and reactions. Remember, mindset/framing plays a big part in how much tension is created during times of diabetes burnout.

Finding Community

Each person's experience with diabetes is different, but sharing frustration, anger, challenges, and sadness with others who can truly relate helps reduce the pressure and stress of living with diabetes. Today, people can get connected to others with diabetes through channels that work for a range of personalities, schedules, and lifestyles (see Chapter 8: Resource Guide on page 195). You can help your loved one find a diabetes community (D-community), blog, or individual source that is a good fit. You can even find posts of people sharing their experience with diabetes burnout and what they do to get through it.

➤ **In person:** Most communities have support groups that meet regularly for people living with diabetes.

Check with the local hospital systems in your loved one's community or with his or her health care provider to find one nearby. If there is nothing close or convenient, see if your loved one might be interested in starting a peer group in the area. Also consider starting a group for yourself and other people living "near" diabetes. Remember, *you* deserve support, too!

➤ **Online:** If in-person group meetings are difficult to make or are uncomfortable, try finding online forums, websites, and blogs. The online world is full of people sharing their experiences, successes, and frustrations concerning life with diabetes. Spend some time looking online to find a group, blog, or individual that "speaks" to your loved one's life with diabetes. A word of caution regarding online sites: while they are an excellent way to feel connected and supported, they should not be seen as a source for medical advice or information. Please always have your loved one check with a health care provider about any medical advice or recommendations.

Whether your loved one chooses to be an active or passive participant, being part of the D-community helps people get through periods of burnout.

How Can *You* Help?

Offer Help That Is . . . Helpful

Even loved ones with the best intentions can get under a person's skin when it comes to diabetes. Make sure you're asking what you can do that would be helpful to them. Think about your loved one's most dreaded task(s) related to diabetes.

Counting carbs? Dealing with insurance? Keeping a logbook? Answering questions about it? Whatever it is, offer to give him or her a break and take that task over for a week or more. (Sorry, but blood glucose checks still have to come from your loved one's fingers!) Being able to take a partial diabetes vacation without the guilt and ramifications of neglecting important diabetes tasks can go a long way toward helping someone through phases of burnout.

☐ **SECRET STRATEGY #4**
· ·
To help alleviate burnout, offer to temporarily take over a diabetes-related task that your loved one particularly dislikes.

Get Moving, Together

Offer to do an activity with your loved one that you both enjoy. We're not suggesting going to the gym together 6 days a week only to be disappointed when you don't make it that often. Instead, try for doing 15–30 minutes of walking, dancing, gardening, playing with the dog, riding a bike, or doing yoga . . . anything that relieves stress and builds a feeling of optimism and empowerment. Doing activities together makes them more fun and is beneficial for you both!

Have Realistic Expectations

Good diabetes management is not perfect diabetes management. Sometimes the pressure to get it right all of the time is at the root of burnout for your loved one with diabetes. Because it is *impossible* to achieve perfect blood glucose control, striving for perfect blood glucose control sets up repeated failure. As humans, we want to avoid things that we perceive we don't do well. Hence, if every blood glucose reading outside of target range is seen as failure, or we beat ourselves up every time we neglect some aspect of diabetes management, it can lead to a common burnout behavior: avoidance of diabetes tasks altogether. You can help your loved one avoid the perfectionism trap by reinforcing messages that diabetes won't go right all the time, and that's OK.

Find a diabetes health care provider/educator who understands this, too, and who will work to establish healthy, realistic diabetes goals and plans. You can help your loved one view a diabetes plan as a roadmap and not as a scorecard of success or failure. You can help reinforce the understanding with your loved one that diabetes will always have its ups and downs and empathize when things don't go as planned.

Seek Professional Help

Burnout may have an accomplice: depression. Depression is a reality for approximately 19 million Americans with and without diabetes. Whether depression is the cause or the result of diabetes burnout, leaving it untreated greatly increases the likelihood that burnout will persist or progress. Ask your health care provider for recommendations for someone who can help you with your depression.

Hello—What About You?

Very much like diabetes burnout, parents, partners, and other support people can experience caregiver fatigue and burnout. Often, it's difficult for people experiencing caregiver fatigue to realize it until they themselves become ill or they hit an emotional/physical wall and simply can't provide care anymore. The statements below can help you know if you're experiencing caregiver fatigue and are at risk of burnout. The more statements that apply to you, the greater the likelihood that you're experiencing caregiver fatigue or burnout.

➤ It's hard for me to find time to do the things I enjoy doing.

➤ I have trouble sleeping at night and often wake up tired.

➤ I feel I have lost touch with my friends and other social networks.

➤ I have annoying physical problem(s).

➤ I know exercise is good for me, but I can't find the time to do it.

➤ There are days when I feel trapped.

➤ I feel guilty that I resent my caregiver responsibilities.

➤ I hesitate to ask family or friends for help because I don't want to burden them.

If many of these statements apply to you, it's time to start focusing on helping yourself . . . not tomorrow, not next week, not next month, but today! Taking care of yourself isn't selfish. It benefits you and everyone around you. Here are steps to relieve symptoms of caregiver fatigue.

Secure Your Mask First Before Helping Others!

Anyone who has flown on a plane has heard this phrase. You *must* make yourself a priority because you are important. You have heard about the importance of eating right, exercising, managing stress, and getting enough sleep a hundred times. The reason you've heard this so often is because these actions are the key ingredients to physical and emotional health. These common sense measures need to be at the top of your list for self-care.

Take time to look closely at each of these areas (eating, exercise, stress, sleep) and identify what you will do to make sure you are able to get what you need. This step likely involves asking for help. Perhaps this is not your style, but ask anyway!

Some of the strategies to overcome/prevent caregiver burnout are the same ones that address diabetes burnout. There is a power in community and peer support for caregivers, so reread Finding Community earlier in this chapter while thinking about things that you will do for yourself. Additionally, here are strategies and resources that are specific to addressing the unique needs of caregivers.

Strategies to Combat Caregiver Fatigue

Value Yourself

There is an interesting (not fair, but interesting) dynamic that can come into play for chronic-condition caregivers. Sometimes there is an inverse relationship between the amount/duration of support you give and the amount of appreciation you receive for giving that support and sacrifice. Translated: the more you do, the less you're appreciated. Have you felt this way before?

FACTOID #9

The more you give, the less you may be appreciated.

Consider these realities:

➤ Age or other circumstances may prevent your loved one from being capable of understanding how much you are doing or sacrificing on his or her behalf.

➤ When your loved one with diabetes stops tending to diabetes responsibilities because you have "taken over," he or she soon forgets the amount of work and sacrifice that goes into it.

➤ Family members and friends may resent the fact that your care for the person with diabetes takes away from time for/with them.

➤ Employers might be understanding at the beginning of a crisis, but over time, that fades. If your caregiving responsibilities interfere with your ability to do your job, it becomes a problem for your employer.

It's likely that as time goes on, your caregiving may even receive criticism rather than praise from others. That is why it is critical that you practice self-praise and learn to truly value yourself and what you do. One way to help you do this is to think about what it would take for someone to replace you, or think about how much you would appreciate it if someone provided *you* with the same loving care. Above all, value yourself by finding ways to make time to meet your needs.

Set Boundaries

If you are overextended as a caregiver, it could be that you're also out of balance with other areas of family life, work, school, and in the community. You may be either giving too much or neglecting certain areas. Now is the time to carefully assess everything on your plate. Audit the things that you've taken on and ask yourself these questions:

➤ Am I doing this out of guilt or a false sense of obligation?

➤ Does this really have to be me, or can someone else do it?

➤ Am I doing more than my fair share because I'm willing to do so?

➤ Am I doing this because I think or others think I "should" do it?

➤ Is my time as a caretaker taking over my ability to be involved in other important relationships?

Use the answers to these questions to help you realign where you're spending your time, and remove or reduce the things you're doing just because you think you "should" do them. With the new bandwidth you've created, add in activities that nurture *your* mind, body, and spirit.

Here are some examples of self-nurturing activities:

➤ Sign up for a class that interests you.

➤ Find a walking buddy and take regular walks.

➤ Spend time in nature or an artistic setting (parks, trails, museums, or a hip part of town).

➤ Reconnect with friends and family with whom you've fallen out of touch.

Share the Load

It's common in diabetes households for one person to take on the majority of the diabetes tasks. A number of things encourage the role of *default diabetes owner* such as primary caregiver status, personality, captain of the kitchen, previous knowledge or skills, guilt, or desire for control. Regardless of what earns you that role, the result is usually the same. The "responsible party" views diabetes management as his or her responsibility. It's up to this person to make sure supplies are never forgotten, doctor's appointments are made, prescriptions are filled, and carbs are counted, calculated, and recorded.

Life alongside diabetes is a marathon. To avoid exhaustion and collapse, it's helpful to set up routines that support the long-term process rather than just the short-term needs.

If there are multiple people who can contribute to diabetes management tasks, approach diabetes as a family affair. Even young siblings can play a role by being responsible for certain tasks like recording numbers in logs or letting someone know when juice boxes are running low.

SECRET STRATEGY #5

Spreading the responsibilities over several family members helps you to avoid burnout and makes everyone feel more involved.

Diabetes management offers more than enough to go around! Spreading the love, if you will, accomplishes three major things. First, it makes the workload of diabetes more manageable for everyone. Second, it gives other family members the ability to contribute, which, in turn, relieves their sense of helplessness. Last, but definitely not least, it makes the person with diabetes feel supported and gives the sense that he or she isn't going it alone.

Asking for Help: Tips and Conversation Starters

Tips

➤ Recognize that people feel good when they are needed. Most friends, neighbors, and family members would love to help, but they don't know how to offer help without coming across as "butting in."

➤ Depending on other people deepens your bond and level of intimacy. Whether it's your friend, sister, or partner, showing vulnerability makes you human and is the foundation for intimate relationships. You may feel like you are protecting a relationship by not burdening the ones you love, but this actually can be a barrier to closeness.

CASE STUDY
. . . .

Here's a real-life example that shows how one family is truly making diabetes a family affair. The family unit consists of the mom, grandparents, a 3-year-old boy, and a 5-year-old girl with type 1 diabetes. In this family, the mom is definitely the primary caregiver; however, she's getting lots of support from family members.

The grandfather picks the kids up from preschool, and the grandmother takes care of lunch and watches them for the afternoon. In this family, the mom and the grandmother have worked together, so that the grandmother could learn how to give insulin through the pump, count carbs, and check blood glucose levels. She also understands when and how to treat a low blood glucose level.

The grandfather considers himself a technical wiz and downloads information from the pump, reviews numbers, comes to doctor's appointments, and makes trips to the pharmacy. Although the 3-year-old brother is a little young for most tasks, he's been reported to faithfully show up with his sister's favorite stuffed animal when it's time to change her pump infusion set, which is her least favorite part of diabetes.

We recognize not every family has grandparents or other relatives who live close enough to be this involved in daily care. But often the real barrier to having this type of support doesn't come from lack of available people, but rather with a discomfort in asking for help or releasing control. Releasing control can be especially hard when it comes to the health and well-being of loved ones.

Conversation Starters

➤ I like the way you organize *XYZ*; do you think you could help me organize all this insurance information and prescriptions?

➤ Lately, I haven't been able to find time to exercise, and I really need to. Would you be willing to do the morning check and dosing on Tuesdays and Thursdays so I can walk with my friend?

➤ If I teach you what you need to know, would you be willing to take care of *Julie* from time to time? I could really use a break every once in a while.

Because most of you reading this book are not looking for self-care tips, note that these same conversation starters can be turned around to offer help to your loved one with diabetes.

➤ I love to organize. Would you like me to help organize your insurance and prescription information?

➤ I know how busy you are. I'm happy to take the kids to school on Tuesdays and Thursdays so you can meet your friend for walks.

➤ I know diabetes can be a lot of work. What do you think about teaching me how to download your pump so I can help run reports to get ready for your doctor's appointments?

When Is It More Than Burnout?

Depression is more than just a bout of the blues and is different from diabetes distress or burnout. This condition isn't a weakness and you can't simply "snap out of it." Depression

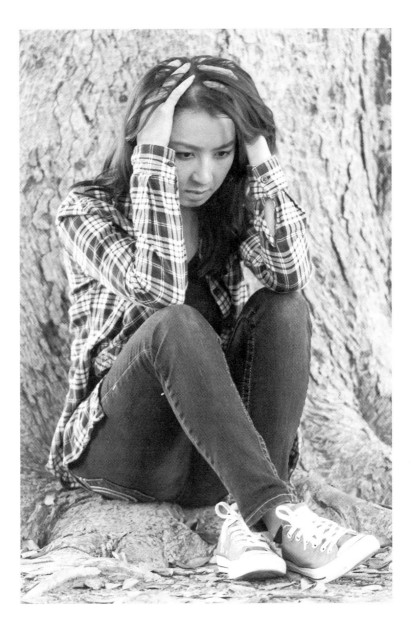

may come and go for some people, while others may be chronically depressed. Some people may require long-term treatment, while others improve with short-term treatment. Most people with depression feel better with medication, talk therapy, or both.

FACTOID #10

Depression is a mood disorder that causes a persistent feeling of sadness and loss of interest. Also called "major depressive disorder" or "clinical depression," it affects how you feel, think, and behave and can lead to a variety of emotional and physical problems. A person experiencing depression may have trouble doing normal day-to-day activities and may sometimes feel as if life isn't worth living.

According to the National Institute of Mental Health, symptoms of depression include the following:

➤ Difficulty concentrating, remembering details, and making decisions

➤ Fatigue and decreased energy

➤ Feelings of guilt, worthlessness, and/or helplessness

➤ Feelings of hopelessness and/or pessimism

➤ Insomnia, early-morning wakefulness, or excessive sleeping

➤ Irritability or restlessness

➤ Loss of interest in activities or hobbies once pleasurable, including sex

➤ Overeating or appetite loss

➤ Persistent aches or pains, headaches, cramps, or digestive problems that do not ease even with treatment

➤ Persistent sad, anxious, or "empty" feelings

➤ Thoughts of suicide or suicide attempts

Depression can be a barrier to healthy eating, exercise, and even basic personal hygiene. Knowing this makes it easier to see how someone experiencing depression might also lose his or her ability to maintain diabetes care routines.

Definition of Anxiety and Panic Attacks

Anxiety disorder is fairly common and is defined by feelings of uneasiness, worry, and fear. While everyone experiences some degree of anxiety from time to time, a person with an anxiety disorder feels an excessive amount of anxiety to the point that it becomes disruptive to daily life.

Panic attacks are the physical manifestation of intense anxiety. They are defined as a sudden and intense attack of anxiety that includes feelings of impending danger, trembling, sweating, pounding heart, and other physical symptoms.

For people living with diabetes, there are certain topics or situations that may trigger anxiety or panic attacks such as "going low," driving, unfamiliar foods, needles, nighttime lows, travel/being away from home or caregivers, new environments, or new work situations.

It's important to understand that concerns about these situations are founded on actual increased levels of risk. The fact is, having a low blood glucose reaction at night or while driving does put a person at risk. Well-meaning efforts to minimize the likelihood of something bad happening don't work and often leave the person with diabetes feeling misunderstood and/or that they are "crazy."

An experienced professional will work with the person to channel the mind's protective signals into productive strategies. This redirection of energy and focus interrupts the escalating level of worry while still addressing the very real safety concern.

CASE STUDY
· · · · · · · · ·

Lynn is a 26-year-old woman who has had type 1 diabetes since she was 12. Growing up, Lynn didn't want to deal with diabetes and frequently skipped taking insulin at mealtime and didn't pay much attention to counting carbs and how much insulin she was dosing.

One time in her late teens, Lynn reversed her long-acting and mealtime insulin and accidentally gave herself 14 units of fast-acting insulin thinking it was long-acting insulin. Lynn realized what had happened shortly after she first went low and was able to treat the situation by eating enough food over the next few hours to cover the insulin.

Even though Lynn effectively managed the situation without suffering any serious immediate consequences, the lasting effect was that Lynn developed severe anxiety related to giving herself insulin. This anxiety showed up in that she was unable to give herself more than 3 units of insulin at any one time. As a result, her blood glucose levels were very high throughout her teen years.

Her high A1C and blood glucose levels were a source of a great deal of conflict between her and her parents. Her doctor kept telling her how important it was that she manage her diabetes and eventually told her parents that, if she wasn't going to be compliant, there was nothing they could do to improve her glucose levels.

(continues)

CASE STUDY (*Continued*)
. . . .

As a young adult, Lynn became concerned for her health and wanted to keep her blood glucose in range. Because she had not addressed her underlying anxiety related to overdosing on insulin, she started restricting her food as a way to manage blood glucose. While this did lower her blood glucose, it created a situation where Lynn would only eat a limited variety of foods and wouldn't eat at all if she was away from home or wasn't 100% sure she knew how many carbs the food contained.

Feeling increasingly unhappy and concerned with her anxiety level, Lynn started going to therapy to address her anxiety issues. With the help of counseling, Lynn addressed her anxiety and is now able to give herself the amount of insulin necessary to cover a balanced meal, and she rarely restricts her food choices to avoid insulin.

Depression, anxiety, and panic attacks are closely related and should be treated by a qualified health care professional. There have been many advances in the treatment of depression and anxiety. Today, treatment options include talk therapy, medication, and/or homeopathic and holistic therapies. Treatment of depression may take some time and trial and error to find what works best. It's important to find a qualified provider to lead the process. Don't be discouraged if the first attempt at treatment isn't successful.

A word of caution
People with untreated depression or anxiety often self-medicate with alcohol or drugs. In cases where someone is using a substance to self-medicate, the substance use must be addressed first before other treatment options will be

effective. Alcohol, which many think of as a stimulant, is actually a depressant and can make depression worse.

FACTOID #11

Although many people think alcohol is a stimulant, it's actually a depressant.

Disordered Eating, Eating Disorders, and Diabulimia

Diabetes comes with a continual focus on food: when to eat, what to eat, how much to eat. It's no wonder that people with diabetes are at a greater risk of developing unhealthy or disordered eating habits. This is particularly true for women. A study done at the Joslin Diabetes Center in Boston, Massachusetts, reported that women with type 1 diabetes are more than twice as likely to develop an eating disorder as women of the same age without diabetes.

Although they sound similar, disordered eating and an eating disorder are not the same thing. With an **eating disorder**, food intake and weight issues consume your thoughts and actions, making it nearly impossible to focus on anything else. Eating disorders often cause multiple, serious physical problems and, in severe cases, can become life-threatening. On the other hand, **disordered eating** is much more common. Disordered eating can be defined as an unhealthy relationship with food, whereas an eating disorder is a psychiatric illness that has a more complex origin and treatment requirement.

Although both conditions are cause for concern, there are signs to look for to know whether someone has disordered eating or an eating disorder. Red flags for both include:

➤ Restrictive dieting/skipping meals: not eating if blood glucose is above a certain level, only eating limited food items, or severely limiting the amount of food eaten

➤ Binging: uncontrolled, excessive eating at a single session, well past the point of fullness

➤ Purging: using vomiting or laxatives to eliminate food intake after meals

➤ Laxatives/diet pill abuse

The behaviors above suggest that a person has developed an unhealthy relationship with food and/or has unhealthy eating habits. However, when combined with the following symptoms, the person may have developed an eating disorder:

➤ Withdrawing from social activities

➤ Distorted body image (thinks they are overweight when they aren't)

➤ Persistent concern about being "fat"

➤ Frequently checking themselves in the mirror

➤ Feeling ashamed, sad, or anxious

➤ Obsessive thinking about food, weight, or shape

➤ Compulsive activity such as counting bites of food, repeatedly weighing or measuring food, eating a limited variety of foods, or eating the exact same foods at the exact time all the time

Diabulimia

Diabulimia is an eating disorder that is specific to people with type 1 diabetes. From a psychological standpoint, diabulimia is similar to bulimia or anorexia in that there is an unhealthy obsession with body image and desire to lose weight. What makes this condition unique to people with diabetes is that people with diabulimia use insulin manipulation to cause weight loss. Simply put, insulin deprivation causes people to lose weight.

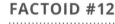

FACTOID #12

> People with diabulimia use insulin manipulation to cause weight loss.

Early signs and symptoms of diabulimia include:

➤ Extremely high A1C results

➤ Blood glucose levels that vary widely for no known reason

➤ Unusual fear of being weighed

➤ Delayed puberty, lack of age-appropriate menstruation, irregular menstruation

➤ Recurring severe low blood glucose events

➤ Obsessive exercising

➤ Food and/or alcohol binges

Treatment for diabulimia is similar to treatment for anorexia and bulimia and includes nutritional counseling and cognitive behavioral therapy to modify beliefs related to weight, eating habits, and insulin use. Depending on the severity of the case, the person may need to be hospitalized. Because insulin is being used to create weight loss, treatment for diabulimia is a highly specialized field and requires a multidisciplinary team to treat it safely and effectively. See specific resources in Chapter 8.

KEY POINTS

➤ People spend varying amounts of time in each stage of grief and may skip or repeat a stage.

➤ Emotional health has a significant impact on physical health.

➤ Diabetes burnout is very common. But sometimes it's more than burnout and may be depression.

➤ People with diabetes are at increased risk for depression, anxiety, and disordered eating.

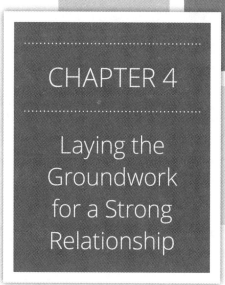

CHAPTER 4

Laying the Groundwork for a Strong Relationship

Now that you're familiar with the ABCs of the physical and emotional aspects of diabetes, let's look at what happens when all of these moving parts leave the doctor's office and are pushed out into the real world.

As part of the support team, you'll need some solid "insider information" to get an idea of what to expect, when to lean in and when to lean out, what is helpful, and what has the potential to create conflict. So, how do you support a person with diabetes without eroding your relationship?

Because effective communication is at the root of all successful relationships, it's probably no surprise that we're going to devote a significant section of this book to that very subject.

....

Diabetes and Relationships:
Real Quotes from Real People

What is it like to have a loved one with diabetes?

"Sometimes it stinks because he gets more attention at night."

– 6-year-old sibling to older brother with diabetes

"I feel bad at site changes because I know she doesn't like it and she has to do it all the time."

– Grandmother to 5-year-old child with diabetes

"I know she hates diabetes so I try to help; I can always tell when she's low and needs to test."

– Best friend to a 12-year-old girl with diabetes

"I feel like I never know what to cook anymore; everything seems to raise his blood glucose."

– Spouse of a person with diabetes

"I wish I had a thing (CGM) that went bee-do bee-do at night, and mom would come into my room. It's not fair; he gets to see her at night, and I don't."

– 4-year-old sibling

"I wish my son knew that I sometimes forget how hard it must be to have a disease that is always there; that is a constant challenge. This disease has taken away some of the carefree aspects of his childhood. When

I am burned out from the midnight blood checks or the unexpected trips to the nurse's office at school, I remind myself that he never lets type 1 slow him down or knock him down. His bravery and strength seem to be endless."

– Mom to 10-year-old son with type 1 diabetes

What do you want your loved one(s) to know about diabetes?

"I wish my family understood that I never forget that I have diabetes; it's just that sometimes I wish I could."

– Person with diabetes for 12 years

"I might not talk about it much, but I think about it all the time."

– Person with diabetes for 30 years

"It's not so bad; it's a pain, but it really is OK, and I'm OK."

– 32-year-old adult with diabetes

Communication and Support

Finding the sweet spot between being helpful and supportive and being overbearing and intrusive is the Holy Grail of a successful diabetes partnership. Feelings such as fear, anger, guilt, and worry can override our internal gauge that would normally help us navigate toward a comfortable balance between nag and support.

Whether your loved one with diabetes is an adult or a child, knowing that diabetes is a serious condition with serious health implications creates the strong need to fix and control things. For decades, the push to "fix and control" diabetes has greatly influenced the behavior of health care providers, scientists, caregivers, and even the general public, and people with diabetes often come away feeling attacked and full of shame. This cloud can set the stage for unproductive relationships on the topic of diabetes.

The fact that you're reading this book says that you don't want your diabetes relationship to feel like a battleground. You're looking for more effective ways to help your loved one with diabetes live a healthy, happy life, and you want to feel more comfortable and confident in your role as diabetes copilot. This is a pretty big topic, so we've broken it down into a few key principles.

Principle 1: Human Before Diabetes; Human After Diabetes

Sounds obvious, but this principle often gets overlooked. The person with diabetes is still the same person as before developing diabetes, complete with personality traits, strengths, weaknesses, and peculiarities. Use this principle to determine which communication approaches will be effective and which won't. Recognize that one size does not fit all!

The good news is that what works well for other areas of your relationship will likely work for issues related to diabetes. For example, consider the following:

➤ Do you and your loved one work well together in a crisis or under stress?

➤ Do you have effective ways to talk about difficult topics?

➤ Do you have open communication where you are able to share your needs and frustrations?

Diabetes has the ability to shine a light (a very bright light) on areas of your relationship that need attention. Improving these rough spots will likely require new approaches. The good news is, when you get it right on diabetes issues, that success will carry over to other areas of your relationship as well. That is a nice bonus!

If you and your loved one already have success sharing tasks, navigating personal boundaries, and working through challenges, you'll be able to apply those same approaches to the diabetes domain.

At the heart of this principle is acknowledging that diabetes is something that gets *added* to a person's life. It doesn't replace the person (or the relationship) you knew before diabetes. Many people (including health care professionals) have the expectation that once a person has diabetes, he or she will (or should) become a completely new person with different organizational skills, communication styles, eating habits, attention to detail, aptitude for numbers, beliefs toward medicine, thresholds for pain, and so on. Read this want ad, and we think you'll get the point.

Wanted

Person with impeccable time management and organization skills, capable of synthesizing large amounts of data at all hours of the day/night. Ability to multitask is essential. Candidate will be asked to perform math calculations, minor surgical procedures, and deliver both rescue and maintenance treatments at all hours of the day and night.

Candidate must be comfortable dealing with life and death situations and have a high threshold for physical discomfort. Candidate will have strong

(continues)

Wanted (*Continued*)

command of macronutrients, meal composition, human pathophysiology, and medication action and interactions.

Position offers no pay, and 24/7/365 attendance is mandatory. Ideally, the candidate will be obsessive-compulsive and able to stick to tight regimens while maintaining a carefree, low-stress lifestyle. Coworkers will offer frequent suggestions to improve your performance and greatly appreciate that you have a sunny disposition and positive work attitude while performing your duties. Apply here.

Crazy, right? But the reality is that diabetes *is* a 24/7 365-day job that requires skills across a wide range of areas with few tangible rewards. Do you know someone who is an amazing organizer? Communicates effectively? Works well with technology? Analyzes numbers and information quickly? Is naturally high-energy, with healthy habits? How many people can you name who have *all* of those attributes? Diabetes management is asking for just such a person. It's no wonder so many people living with diabetes have periods when they feel like failures.

Principle 2: Perfect Diabetes Management Is a Myth

Not only is perfect diabetes management not obtainable, it simply doesn't exist—no matter the person or the effort. Once that reality is on the table, you can spend time matching diabetes skill requirements to skillsets for both you and your loved one. This process will become the cornerstone of building an effective and enjoyable diabetes partnership. With diabetes care tasks aligned with natural strengths, and gaps in skills identified, you and your loved one can build a highly successful plan for diabetes management.

Principle 3: Words Matter

The importance and power of words is in no way limited to the topic of diabetes. Minds greater than ours have shown that what we hear, say, and think has a direct impact on how we feel—emotionally and physically—as well as what we can achieve. Well-known author Dr. Wayne Dyer states in his book *Power of Intention,* "What you're feeling is a function of how you're thinking and what you're saying."

The root of this principle is word dynamics: *word →* *thoughts → manifestation.* The words that we hear and choose become part of our belief system and then contribute greatly to our reality. For example, if we think and believe that we will fail at something, our likelihood of failing is greatly increased. If we focus our energy on thinking we're sick or that we're getting sick, our immune system is weakened and we increase our likelihood of getting sick.

We (unknowingly) seek to create alignment between what we believe and what we see as reality. Therefore, if we believe we are failures at something, our subconscious will look for information that supports that belief. This in turn makes the belief stronger and gives it more momentum to influence outcomes.

So how does this all relate to diabetes? Diabetes touches our lives throughout the day, every day. There are *countless* times that we use or hear words that refer to some aspect of life with diabetes. The words that we choose will influence how we and our loved ones feel. They can make us feel like a victim, helpless, blamed, and full of shame, or they can make us feel proud, capable, and empowered to take charge of our health.

Let's start by looking at the word "empowerment." It would be ridiculous to hope for a person to be happy about diabetes (why should anyone be happy about the burdens and risks that come with diabetes?). However, if a person feels *empowered*, they will have a greater sense of well-being and will likely take steps to fit diabetes into their lives.

For people living with diabetes, the messages that come from health care teams, loved ones, the general public, and ultimately themselves are full of words like "good," "bad," "should," "control," "diabetic," "adherence," and "compliance." All of these are words are used to talk about and evaluate (judge) how people with diabetes are handling diabetes management. These words are often combined with other words to send even stronger messages: **good adherence, poor control, should eat right, won't test blood glucose, has bad numbers, has good control**, as well as **he is, she isn't, they are**, or **he has**. See where we're going with this? "He is a good diabetic." "She is poorly controlled." "You should follow the doctor's plan."

Diabetes is a chronic condition that comes with a great deal of blame, shame, guilt, and misunderstanding about what it is and how it "should" be treated. Using terms like the ones above foster feelings of failure and the belief that the person with diabetes is to blame for poor diabetes "control."

Let's face it . . . no one wants to get a "bad" score on a test. That's true of your blood glucose "test" as well. If we think of blood glucose numbers as tests that have good or bad scores, the person with diabetes is being set up for judgment by themselves and others. However, when we use language that supports the reality that blood glucose readings are information that can be used to make better decisions, a sense of empowerment and confidence is gained. It is comforting to know that no number is good or bad as long as we can use the information it represents to our benefit.

Sample Word Swaps

Defeating Term	Empowering Term	Message Shift
Diabetic	Has or lives with diabetes	The person **is** diabetes → the person **has** diabetes
Good/bad blood glucose	Above/below/within target range	Success/failure → requires action/ doesn't require action
Control	Management	Suggests perfect is possible → recognizes it's a process with varying results
Adherence/ compliance	Treatment barriers	Viewing person with diabetes as the problem → identifying factors affecting effectiveness of diabetes treatment plan
Blood glucose test	Blood glucose check	Judgment or score of performance → touch point to see if action is needed
Disease	Condition	The person is sick → the person has a condition that requires management

Remember our discussion in the previous chapter about "framing"? Word choices play an important role in helping us reframe situations. If we view (frame) a person with diabetes as "sick," our response is probably going to be that the person needs to be "taken care of." Conversely, if we view the person with diabetes as having a condition that needs management (and a lot of it!), our response is more likely to focus on how we can help him or her to better manage. This small shift in framing has a dramatic impact on how you treat and interact with your loved one with diabetes. And for the person with diabetes, being supported feels very different than being taken care of and feeling like you're unable to take care of yourself.

SECRET STRATEGY #6

Reframing "taking care of" to "supporting" enforces the understanding that you cannot control another person, nor should you try. However, you can and should support self-care, individualization, and empowerment.

Principle 4: Have Realistic Expectations for Yourself and Your Loved One with Diabetes

➤ It is not necessary to be perfect. Your loved one isn't going to have perfect blood glucose levels, and you are not going to always remember to refrain from nagging about diabetes management.

➤ Diabetes doesn't take a vacation, but people do. For different reasons, and at different times, people with diabetes may relax (drop) their diabetes tasks. This is common and to be expected.

➤ Recognize the ebb and flow. What's happening now isn't necessarily permanent. Just because things seem hectic or chaotic around diabetes, doesn't mean it will always be this way. The same is true in reverse. Don't panic if someone you love suddenly seems to be struggling with diabetes. Diabetes and how people cope with diabetes can change as other areas of life change.

➤ Understand (and accept) how milestone events will affect diabetes management and adjust accordingly.

➤ Interest in doing diabetes tasks won't always peak at the same time. You know how it is when a topic grabs your interest (a good book, exercise, or a new project at work) or something motivates you to invest more energy than usual into an area. Don't assume that because you read a compelling article on the positive effects of exercise on diabetes that your loved one will share your excitement or motivation.

➤ Forgive yourself for nagging. Despite your best intentions, it will happen sometimes!

Putting It All Together for a Smoother Ride

With these key principles and dynamics of communication addressed, you can begin to create effective relationship strategies and action plans. The goal is to build a system for communication and support that incorporates your need for peace of mind and your loved one's need for actual *peace*. People can fall into the trap of assuming the other person understands their needs and that the person sees things with the same urgency and importance. Avoid that trap . . . don't assume! Have a conversation about how you and your loved one will talk about diabetes.

You could open a conversation with something like this: "Look, I know it drives you crazy when I constantly ask you about diabetes. But I love you, and it drives me crazy to think that you might be in danger. Can we sit down and figure out what would work for both of us?" It is fine to include feelings and emotions in the discussion, but the focus of this conversation should be on developing a plan rather than venting emotions. When there's an argument or tension, there's usually two sides (at least) to what people are experiencing. Here are the two sides of common situations when it comes to life with diabetes:

➤ You're always asking what my number is/You never tell me what your numbers are.

➤ It drives me crazy when you constantly ask if I checked my glucose level/When I don't know where your blood glucose level is, I worry that you'll have a low.

➤ I should be able to decide what to eat and when/I'm afraid that if you eat certain foods your diabetes will get worse.

➤ I get sick of always talking about diabetes/I worry that you aren't managing your diabetes.

In many families and relationships, diabetes takes center stage and sucks up too much energy. Yes, we all want to make sure that we are doing everything we can to minimize the health risks associated with diabetes, but you and your loved one deserve to be the focus of your lives . . . **not diabetes**.

So how do you place diabetes in the background of your relationship without ignoring it or denying that it exists? The first step is to make it a habit to always acknowledge the *person* before the diabetes. For example, have the first thing you say in the morning, or after school, or when returning from work, be something about the person. An example would be, "How did you sleep?" or "Good morning" instead of "What's your number?" or some other diabetes question. Except for situations where the person needs immediate attention, such as when having a low blood glucose reaction, the business of diabetes can wait.

For instance, why do you need to ask your loved one for his or her blood glucose number in the morning? You might answer, "I'm the one who makes breakfast, and I need to know if the number is high so I know what to make. I try not to make pancakes or oatmeal on high mornings because I know these foods will make blood glucose levels even higher." In this scenario, it seems like you need to know the morning number. But what if the two of you worked out a system that on mornings when the reading is high you make eggs and Canadian bacon instead of oatmeal or pancakes.

So what you really need to know is, "What am I making for breakfast?" By having the pre-conversation about the plan for high blood glucose mornings, your morning conversation could now sound like this:

YOU   "Good morning. Did you have a good night? What would you like for breakfast?"

YOUR LOVED ONE "I slept pretty well. Eggs would be great. Thanks."

And just like that, diabetes is factored into the morning routine without being brought into the limelight. From a food perspective, the high blood glucose is being addressed. For a single blood glucose reading, there's no reason to dwell on the why, where, and what of it. Just treat it, or make related decisions and move on. No shame, no blame, no guilt. Through pre-conversations about the cause and effect of morning blood glucose numbers and breakfast selection, you've addressed diabetes ahead of time, so now it doesn't have to be part of the discussion each and every morning.

Diabetes is an important topic that permeates so many parts of our lives, and not every exchange between you and your loved one can (or should) be completely diabetes-free. But by simply being mindful about what and when you're asking about diabetes, and checking to see if there's other information that solves your "need to know," you can reduce the focus and energy that you channel into the diabetes piece of your relationship.

Building a Communication Plan

What goes into a diabetes communication plan? Here are some concepts to consider:

> ➤ Accept that, ultimately, diabetes is *theirs* to manage
> (barring special conditions such as very young

children or adults who are not able to manage their own care).

➤ Use technology such as remote continuous glucose monitoring to serve as an intermediary. (See text below for more details.)

➤ Decide upfront when and how often blood glucose levels need to be checked and what information needs to be shared.

➤ Find out if your loved one wants you to be involved in the problem-solving part of diabetes management. If so, determine when you will work on it together.

➤ Develop general food and activity plans, with adjustments for special situations and occasions.

Once you and your loved one have *jointly* developed a diabetes communication plan, do your best to stick to it. Even with the best intentions, you may still slip and find yourself asking, "Did you do this? Did you eat that? Why didn't you do . . . ?" once in a while. That's OK; you are only expressing your love and concern for your loved one. And we're all only human. Don't give up; with effort, habits can be changed. Anyone reading this book probably knows all too well that nagging, scare tactics, and getting LOUDER are strategies that just don't work.

In some situations, particularly for parents of young children and adult children of elderly parents, you may need to know a lot of the details (blood glucose results, food eaten, insulin given, etc.) so that you can be in a position to provide adequate support and supervision. Here's where leveraging technology can make things a whole lot easier on everyone. Today's meters, pumps, continuous glucose monitors (CGMs), and smartphone apps offer ways to automatically share important diabetes information between family, friends, and health care providers. These devices allow the user to log information and generate reports quite easily. Another way to think about communicating diabetes information with family members is to set up text shortcuts: add emojis and make it fun and personal. Here are a few to get you thinking about what your text shortcuts could look like:

✓↓🍎 = I know my blood glucose is low; I checked it already and I have treated it.

♥☺ = Thanks, I love you. Now I can concentrate on work.

If you're not yet an emoji master, ask someone to help you set up shortcuts for your own common diabetes communications (hint: the best person might be the youngest person in your life). Once created, you can send these messages with literally a single button press!

Honey, Where's My . . . ?
(Getting Organized)

Being disorganized can make managing diabetes much more stressful than it needs to be. Given all there is to do and all the supplies that are involved, keeping up with diabetes care can create a great deal of stress—for both you and your loved one. Whether you're on a business trip, family vacation, moving, or just going out to dinner, being prepared and organized can make everything much easier to manage.

If your loved one lives with you, this is an area where you can really help to reduce the stress and burden that comes with living with diabetes. Let's face it; organization isn't everybody's strong suit. Even with the best intentions and effort, some people struggle with organization. So if organization *is* your thing, here's your chance to shine.

Getting organized takes some upfront effort, but setting up systems will quickly become huge time-savers as well as stress-relievers. In other words, it's well worth the investment.

For a practical, handy reference for helping to organize your loved one's "diabetes life," we highly recommend creating a daily diabetes notebook (you can find a fantastic version in *The Complete Diabetes Organizer: Your Guide to a Less Stressful and More Manageable Diabetes Life* by Susan Weiner and Leslie Josel).

Also, have you embraced smartphone technology? Smartphones can be a huge source of organizational efficiency. If you haven't checked out the large number of diabetes-related, organizational apps yet, diabetes could be just the reason to get started. There are apps that can remind you to do everything from ordering supplies to checking your blood glucose to changing your pump's infusion set (see Chapter 8 for resource guides).

Whether you embrace smartphone apps or rely on a notebook and pencil, one of the key principles of organization is *consistency*. Repetition builds habits, and habits reduce the amount of time and energy spent thinking about and doing just about anything.

Organizational Tools

Smartphone: On a smartphone, you can download free apps that will let you scan documents to email to your care team or insurance, take pictures of things you need to reference, set alarms for appointment reminders, store contact information, or track health statistics.

Apps: Sample apps include Genius Scan; pharmacy apps for auto refill and reminders; blood glucose logs/trackers; or food, fitness, and overall wellness trackers (specific names and links are provided in Chapter 8).

Watch: The Apple Watch has alarm features to display blood glucose readings from a CGM, track steps, or show activity and food intake.

Keep a central file or notebook with all key information: Update this notebook twice a year or as things change.

Maintain a dedicated storage area: This area can be anything from a dedicated area of a room, a closet, or a drawer. The idea is to have all supplies that don't require refrigeration in the same area.

Where to Start?

Diabetes Supplies

Supplies can be divided into two groups: those that require refrigeration and those that don't. For things that don't need refrigeration, find a spot in the house that you can dedicate to storing diabetes supplies. If your loved one wears a pump and a CGM, and you order 3 months' worth of supplies at the same time, you might feel like you need a whole room! Stacking things neatly in compartments will help you to conserve space and keep an eye on inventory.

It is helpful to use open shelves (rather than drawers) so you can quickly see when something is running low. When you get new supplies, stack them from the bottom or from the back so you'll continue to use the oldest items first to avoid letting something expire. If you don't have a shelf that you can dedicate, a drawer or a plastic storage bin will work, too. The key is just to keep them all together and neatly sorted.

Medications that require refrigeration should be stored in the door of the refrigerator to reduce the risk of freezing. Again, stack the newest in the back (or on the bottom) so that your loved one will use things in the order they were received. Highlight expiration dates with a red marker. If a package was opened and then put back into the refrigerator, mark the date it was opened. Once a medication has been opened, it will have a certain number of days before it expires—this is sooner than the expiration date on the box. For example, most types of insulin are good for 1 year if refrigerated and left unopened. Once they have been opened, many expire within 28–30 days, but others last up to 56 days. Check the label insert for specific information about expiration and proper storage for all medications.

· · · · · □ **SAFETY TIP**

> Check the package insert of all medications to understand proper storage instructions and expiration information. Even different forms of insulin have different handling instructions.

On-the-Go Supplies

The contents of someone's on-the-go bag will vary from person to person, but usually includes a glucose meter, emergency medications, and fast-acting carbohydrates to treat low blood glucose levels. Keeping these supplies together in the same bag, which is kept in the same place, will reduce the number of times that you arrive at a destination only to realize that your loved one needs to go back and get his or her "kit."

Prescriptions: Tips and Tricks

➤ Each time your loved one visits the diabetes doctor, have the doctor review prescription expiration dates for all of the diabetes medications and supplies and have the doctor write new prescriptions for anything with less than 4 months remaining.

➤ Ask your pharmacy to synchronize refill dates so that there are fewer trips for refills.

➤ Request a 3-month supply of medications where allowed by insurance. The pharmacy can give you a partial fill for the first month to get multiple refill dates synchronized.

➤ Set up mail-order or pharmacy auto-refill and have the pharmacy send you text or email reminders when ready for pickup or delivery. Make sure that any mail-order delivery for insulin or other medications that require refrigeration are shipped in temperature-controlled packaging.

➤ Keep a photo or electronic copy of all prescriptions on your phone so that they can be easily accessed away from home or in the event of hospitalization.

Insurance

➤ Keep a front and back copy of all current insurance cards on a smartphone or photocopied on paper.

➤ Set reminders for premium due dates or set up online auto-pay.

➤ Keep a folder for all out-of-pocket health care–related expenses for tax purposes and flexible spending accounts.

➤ Set a reminder for the open enrollment period (which usually starts on November 1 and runs through January 31). In most cases, during this time period is the only time insurance can be changed without a qualifying life event. Qualifying life events typically include change in employment, marriage/divorce, or birth/adoption of a child.

Supplies to Treat Low Blood Glucose

People who take insulin (once a day or many times a day) or oral medications that stimulate the pancreas to produce more insulin (sulfonylureas and meglitinides) are at risk of hypoglycemia at any time. Be sure to have nonperishable, fast-acting carbohydrate readily available: in the kitchen, at the bedside, or in your car, purse, briefcase, or backpack. When these sources of carbohydrate are used, remember to restock immediately. Even though you don't have diabetes, as someone who spends time with someone who does, it's a good idea for you to have something with you to treat low blood glucose.

When kept in an area with other food and drink, mark these carbohydrates specifically for low-blood-glucose treatment to ensure they will still be there when you need them. Marking these important items makes it easy for anyone to know where to go to grab something to help your loved one deal with low blood glucose and keeps others from accidentally indulging.

Emergency To-Go Kit

You never know when a major catastrophe will take place. For example, hurricanes or wildfire can force you to evacuate your home with little notice. If you live with a loved one with diabetes, work with them to be prepared for an emergency. Have a bag ready to go that has a 2-week supply of everything your loved one needs for diabetes management. Keep this bag in an easily accessible spot. In addition to regular supplies, make sure the bag includes a meter/pump/CGM batteries, charging cables, pump supplies, glucagon, and plenty of carbohydrates. Having this emergency kit ready to go is especially critical for people living with type 1 diabetes.

Remember that test strips, insulin, and many other medications are temperature-sensitive, so the bag shouldn't be kept in the car. Add a brightly colored note on the outside as a reminder to get medications from the refrigerator in the event of an emergency. Consider including an insulin cooling case (such as a Frio pouch) as part of the kit so that you can protect medications from temperature extremes without refrigeration. Hopefully, you and your loved one will go a lifetime without needing to use the emergency kit, so be sure to check expiration dates and swap out batteries regularly. An easy way to remember to check expiration dates and batteries is to do it when smoke detector batteries are checked or whenever you renew your auto or homeowner's insurance policy.

Standards-of-Care Appointments

"Standards of care" is a term used by health care providers to refer to the type and frequency of checkups that people with diabetes are recommended to have to support their overall health. The type and frequency of these visits will depend on the individual, but the appointments typically include eye exams, dental visits, lab work, foot exams, and primary care appointments.

These checkups are an important part of diabetes management and help to identify potential health concerns early. So set reminders for when next appointments are due and record when they took place. If transportation to appointments is an issue, check with the health insurance company. Many companies will cover the cost of transportation to and from medical appointments. Additionally, county and community services are often available.

A person living with diabetes should follow the specific recommendation of the diabetes doctor. Individual frequency and types of visits will vary, but a typical schedule of check-ups will look something like this:

Sample Schedule for Regular Diabetes Checkups

Type of visit	Frequency	Notes
Diabetes doctor	Every 3–6 months	Checking blood pressure, weight, feet, nutrition, medication review, and A1C
Dentist	Every 4–6 months	Diabetes increases the risk of gum disease and tooth decay
Eye exam	Once a year	Should be with an ophthalmologist experienced with issues related to diabetes
Lab work	Once a year	Diabetes/metabolic panel (blood and urine) to check kidney and thyroid function and lipids

Additional appointments with other specialists such as a certified diabetes educator (CDE), nutritionist, or therapist may also be helpful and necessary.

Doctors' Names and Numbers

Write down (paper or electronic) on a single page the names and contact information (phone numbers, email addresses) for all your health care providers. Take a picture with your phone or make copies. Keep one copy at home and one with you or your loved one. Use your smartphone to keep track of this information.

Piecing Together the Insurance Puzzle

Health insurance is one of the most complex aspects of health care. Most people fail to take full advantage of the benefits offered by their health insurance or find it too confusing to figure out what benefits they are or aren't eligible to receive. As a result, many miss out on important medications, appointments, and benefits because of restrictions imposed by their particular plan. Given the importance health insurance plays in the lives of people with diabetes (not to mention the cost!), it helps to have a solid understanding of how your health insurance works. Here are some ways to make sure your loved one is making the most of insurance options.

Basic Insurance Facts

As of 2014, health insurance plans in the U.S., whether sold inside or outside the government's Health Insurance Marketplace, cannot deny coverage, charge more, or refuse to cover treatments because of diabetes (or any other preexisting condition). People who meet certain income requirements may also qualify for help paying their premiums and other costs for plans purchased through the government Health Insurance Marketplace.

Laws related to preexisting exclusion clauses can change over time. Having continuous insurance coverage may protect people with preexisting conditions from having an interruption in insurance coverage. Although there is protection of coverage for preexisting conditions at the time of this publication, unfortunately, it is possible for new laws to be passed that allow insurance coverage to be denied because of preexisting conditions.

Health insurance sold through the Marketplace must cover a set of "essential health benefits." These include:

➤ Doctor office visits

➤ Emergency room services and hospitalization

➤ Pregnancy and newborn care

➤ Mental health and substance abuse services

➤ Prescription drugs

➤ Rehabilitative services and devices

➤ Laboratory services

➤ Preventive services

➤ Chronic disease management

➤ Children's health services (including oral and vision care)

Open enrollment (when you can typically change insurance plans without a qualifying life event) runs from November 1 through January 31. You can access *free* individual assistance to help you choose and enroll in a plan by contacting your state Health Insurance Marketplace or by using the following website: localhelp.healthcare.gov.

Information to Gather Before Choosing a Plan

➤ Coverage of prescriptions (specify the types and brands taken)

➤ Coverage of durable medical goods (preferred brand of meter/test strips, CGM, pumps, pens)

➤ Are existing providers in-network? (using in-network providers results in the lowest copay for visits and highest coverage percentage)

➤ Cost for visits, specialists, emergency room visits, hospitalization, or lab work

➤ Deductible costs (a deductible is how much a member has to pay out-of-pocket before coverage kicks in; it's becoming increasing popular for insurance companies to offer high-deductible plans that require the member to spend $5,000 to $10,000 for health care products/services—in addition to monthly premiums—before receiving any benefits)

Appeals Process: Know Your Rights
If a health insurer refuses to pay a claim or ends coverage, the member has the right to appeal the decision and have it reviewed by a third party. Members can ask the insurance company to reconsider its decision. Insurers have to explain why they've denied a claim or ended coverage. And they have to let you know how to dispute their decisions.

Details about how to use the appeal process can be found at https://www.healthcare.gov/using-marketplace-coverage/ appealing-insurance-company-decisions.

KEY POINTS

➤ Don't ask if you don't really need to know. To minimize the amount of time spent talking about diabetes, be mindful of when you're asking questions just out of habit and when you can get information other ways (electronic logs/histories).

➤ Prepare for points of potential conflict that tend to occur frequently (e.g., asking for blood glucose numbers).

➤ In general, reduce the amount of time you spend talking about diabetes with your loved one.

➤ Identify set time(s) during the week to review logs and problem-solve.

➤ Leverage technology to exchange information in a fast, "noninvasive" way.

➤ Being organized about diabetes supplies and care can save you and your loved one a great deal of time and frustration. Have a 2-week emergency kit ready to go.

➤ Keep important doctor and prescription information on your smartphone.

➤ Insurance coverage is a complex and rapidly changing area. Use resources to help with coverage and support. A good place to start is localhelp.healthcare.gov.

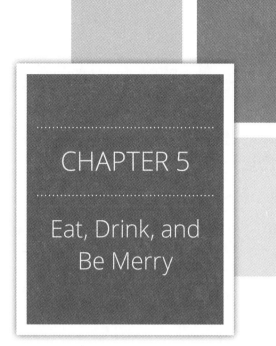

CHAPTER 5

Eat, Drink, and Be Merry

Food is near and dear to many of us. But when living with diabetes, the topic of food can take on a life of its own. If there's tension in your diabetes relationship, there's a very good chance that food is part of it, or perhaps the "main event."

Food plays a key role in diabetes management. Because it's something we partake in several times a day, every day, it can have a huge impact on physical and emotional health. In this chapter, we'll discuss the following:

➤ Nutrition fundamentals

➤ Effects of food on blood glucose

➤ Meal-planning strategies

➤ Mindful eating

➤ Emotional aspects of food for people with diabetes

Much of the information in the chapter is general information and helpful for everyone, whether they are living with diabetes or not. Later in the chapter, we will discuss food and emotions specifically in the context of living with diabetes.

··

Nutrition Fundamentals

There are many types of diets that focus on certain types of food to be included or eliminated—diets such *Paleo, Mediterranean,* or *vegan* are just a few. Rather than a specific diet, this section will talk about the fundamentals of nutrition and healthy meal planning that includes moderate carbohydrate intake, lean protein, healthy fats, fruits, and vegetables. We encourage you and your loved one to meet with a registered dietitian, preferably one who is also a certified diabetes educator, for personalized meal planning.

Macronutrients: Carbohydrates, Protein, and Fats

Carbohydrates

What are carbohydrates? Carbohydrates (or carbs, for short) are the sugars and starches in food that your body breaks down into glucose. They are found in grains, fruits, vegetables, milk products, and sweets.

How do carbs affect blood glucose? Carbohydrates raise blood glucose, and the more simple the form of carbohydrate (sugar, honey, juice), the faster it will raise blood glucose levels.

How should I be thinking about carbs in my diet? Carbohydrates are your body's main source of energy. Not all carbohydrates are created equal. Carbohydrates such as fruits, vegetables, and high-fiber grains give your body the energy and nutritional elements it needs with a slower effect on blood glucose rise. Carbohydrates such as candy, donuts, and sweetened drinks create a significant spike in blood glucose and deliver little or no nutritional value.

Protein

What is protein? Protein is found in chicken, beef, eggs, seafood, beans, nuts, and seeds. Protein builds and maintains lean muscle and can help stabilize blood glucose levels.

How does protein affect blood glucose? Protein contains little or no carbohydrate, so standard serving sizes have a minimal impact on blood glucose and help to stabilize glucose levels.

How should I be thinking about protein in my diet? Lean protein choices support muscle development and contain less saturated fats than higher-fat sources of protein. Combining carbohydrates with protein helps slow the rise of blood glucose.

Fats

What are fats? Fats are a source of fuel for the body and can store energy. Fats provide flavor and texture to food and make you feel satiated (full and satisfied).

How do fats affect blood glucose? When eaten alone, fats will not raise blood glucose. Fats slow the digestion of carbohydrates and delay the appearance of glucose in the bloodstream.

How should I be thinking about fats in my diet? There are many types of fat; some are healthy and others are not.

Monounsaturated fats (found in olive oil, avocados, and nuts) and polyunsaturated fats (found in sunflower oil, seeds, and fatty fish such as salmon) have been shown to **decrease** the risk of heart disease. Trans fats have been shown to increase the risk of heart disease (trans fats are found in foods with "hydrogenated" or "partially hydrogenated" in the ingredients list, e.g., in foods like margarine, baked goods, or crackers).

Meal Planning: Pulling It All Together

Rather than thinking about foods that you can or can't eat, think of grouping foods in categories that tell you where they fall on the nutritional value scale. This step helps you think about how much and how often to include different foods in meals. There are many different approaches to meal planning available. Some people count the amount of carbohydrate in their meals and match their insulin doses to it. Some restrict the portions of carbohydrate they have in each meal and snack. Others choose slower-digesting forms of carbohydrate whenever possible. But what about those who simply want to "eat healthy"—provide a good balance of nutrients while minimizing harmful fats and foods that cause dramatic spikes in blood glucose levels? The example below is an excerpt from The Livongo Meal Plan™—a meal plan that Diane helped develop with the team of nutrition experts at Livongo Health.

Meal Planning Basics: Green, Yellow, and Red Foods

Planning well-balanced meals can seem like a chore. To make meal planning faster, easier, and even enjoyable, we've provided three food lists from which you can mix and match items to create healthy meals.

To take the guesswork out of what goes into a well-balanced meal, we categorized foods as green, yellow, or red. *Green* foods are always allowed. *Yellow* foods offer important nutrients but should be consumed in small amounts. *Red* foods should be eaten rarely, as an occasional treat.

Use the list below as a guide. If there are foods you don't like, don't force yourself to eat them just because they are green foods. Or, try a different preparation—for example, roast broccoli instead of steaming it. Eat for health *and* for pleasure.

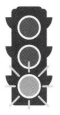

Green Foods

Foods in the green category have little to no effect on blood glucose, provide the most vitamins and minerals, and will fill you up and keep you full throughout the day. Choose these foods most often when planning meals. If you find you are still hungry after a meal and want seconds, these are your go-to foods, since they will satisfy your hunger without causing an additional rise in blood glucose. These are also the best foods to choose when blood glucose is elevated at meal times.

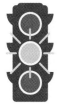

Yellow Foods

Foods in the yellow category are still good choices but are likely to be higher in carbohydrates, which can cause a higher rise in blood glucose. Some of these foods may also be higher in fat. Keep portions from this group small and limit how many servings you include throughout the day.

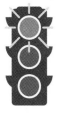

Red Foods

Foods in the red category are high in carbohydrate, high in both saturated and trans fats, or have a low nutritional value. These foods will cause the highest rise in blood glucose after a meal or snack and can cause weight gain. These foods are best eaten as an occasional treat.

Foods to Eat Often (Green Foods), to Eat Daily (Yellow Foods), and to Limit (Red Foods)

Green Foods (Eat Often)	Yellow Foods (Eat Daily)	Red Foods (Limit)
Proteins • Lean beef • Canadian bacon • Chicken without skin • Eggs/egg whites • Fish • Pork • Shellfish • Turkey **Non-Starchy Vegetables** • Asparagus • Beets • Broccoli • Brussels sprouts • Cabbage • Carrots • Cauliflower • Celery • Cucumbers • Eggplant • Green beans • Leafy greens (lettuce, kale, collards, spinach, etc.) • Mushrooms • Okra • Onions • Peppers • Radishes • Snap peas • Tomatoes • Water chestnuts • Yellow squash • Zucchini	**Fruits** • Apples • Applesauce (unsweetened) • Apricots • Bananas • Berries (strawberries, blueberries, blackberries, etc.) • Cherries • Figs • Grapefruit • Grapes • Kiwis • Mangos • Melons (honeydew, cantaloupe, watermelon, etc.) • Nectarines • Oranges • Papaya • Peaches • Pears • Pineapple • Plums **Starchy Vegetables** • Corn • Parsnips • Peas • Potatoes • Sweet potatoes • Squash (acorn, butternut, spaghetti, etc.) • Turnips	**Fruits** • Dried fruits (raisins, dates, etc.) • Frozen fruits w/ added sugar • Fruits canned in syrup **Bread and Grains** • Bagels • Biscuits • Buns (hot dog or hamburger) • Cereal (dry and instant) • Croissants • Muffins • Pancakes • Rolls • Waffles • White flour **Proteins** • Bacon • Beef (regular ground beef, rib roast, pot roast) • Chicken with skin and/or breaded and fried • Chorizo • Hot dogs • Pepperoni • Sausage

(*continues*)

Foods to Eat Often (Green Foods), to Eat Daily (Yellow Foods), and to Limit (Red Foods) (*Continued*)

Green Foods (Eat Often)	Yellow Foods (Eat Daily)	Red Foods (Limit)
Oils and Fats	**Breads and Grains**	**Dairy**

Oils and Fats
- Avocados
- Canola oil
- Olive oil
- Olives

Beverages
- Black coffee (hot or iced)
- Bouillon or broth
- Unsweetened almond or coconut milk
- Unsweetened tea (hot or iced)
- Water (plain, seltzer, sparkling)

Condiments
- Hot sauce (low sodium)
- Mustard
- Salsa
- Sriracha sauce

Seasonings
- Fresh and dried herbs
- Garlic
- Lemon juice
- Lime juice

Breads and Grains
- Barley
- Bread (whole grain preferred)
- Crackers (whole grain preferred)
- Couscous
- English muffins (whole wheat preferred)
- Pasta (whole wheat preferred)
- Pita bread (whole wheat preferred)
- Popcorn (air popped)
- Quinoa
- Rice (brown or wild preferred)
- Steel-cut oats
- Tortillas (corn preferred)

Beans
- Black
- Black-eyed peas
- Garbanzo
- Kidney
- Lentils
- Lima
- Navy
- Pinto
- White

Dairy
- Cheese (processed, American)
- Heavy cream

Beans
- Baked beans
- Refried beans (canned)

Packaged Snacks
- Chips
- Crackers (white)
- Pretzels
- Snack bars
- 100-calorie packs

Sweets and Desserts
- Brownies
- Cakes
- Candy (all)
- Cookies
- Doughnuts
- Frozen yogurt
- Ice cream
- Pastries
- Pie
- Sherbet/sorbet

Beverages
- Alcohol
- Fruit juice/punch
- Lemonade
- Soda/diet soda
- Sports drinks
- Sweetened tea
- Any drink containing sugar

(*continues*)

Foods to Eat Often (Green Foods), to Eat Daily (Yellow Foods), and to Limit (Red Foods) (*Continued*)

Green Foods (Eat Often)	Yellow Foods (Eat Daily)	Red Foods (Limit)
	Dairy	**Oils and Fats**
	▪ Cheese (cheddar, Swiss, provolone, etc.)	▪ Cream cheese
		▪ Margarine
		▪ Shortening
	▪ Cottage cheese	▪ Sour cream
	▪ Greek yogurt (plain)	
	▪ Milk (nonfat or 1% preferred)	**Condiments**
	▪ Rice milk	▪ Agave
	▪ Soy milk (unsweetened)	▪ BBQ sauce
		▪ Honey mustard
	▪ Yogurt (plain or light)	▪ Honey
		▪ Jams/jellies
	Nuts and Seeds	▪ Ketchup
	▪ Almonds	▪ Mayonnaise
	▪ Cashews	▪ Sugar
	▪ Peanuts	▪ Syrup
	▪ Pecans	▪ Teriyaki sauce
	▪ Walnuts	
	▪ Nut butters	
	▪ Seeds (flax, pumpkin, sunflower, etc.)	
	Oils and Fats	
	▪ Butter	
	▪ Coconut oil	
	▪ Peanut oil	
	▪ Safflower oil	
	▪ Sunflower oil	
	▪ Vegetable oil	
	Sweets and Desserts	
	▪ Dark chocolate (72% cocoa and higher)	

Quick Tips for Healthy Eating

➤ **Drink plenty of water.** Early signs of dehydration (headache, dizziness, and feeling tired) are often mistaken for hunger and can lead to unnecessary snacking. Some experts suggest that adults should consume eight to ten 8-ounce glasses of water per day.

➤ **Still hungry after a meal? Eat more non-starchy vegetables.** If you find you want seconds after finishing a meal, eat more non-starchy vegetables like leafy greens, broccoli, and peppers. These foods will have a low effect on your blood glucose, and they contain fiber, which will help you feel fuller faster.

➤ **Keep healthy, low-carb snacks on hand.** Stock up on items like nuts, beef jerky, cut raw vegetables, fruit, and nut butters.

➤ **Plan and prepare meals in advance.** Set aside time each week to wash and chop vegetables, trim and prepare proteins, and cook items like soups and casseroles for the week ahead.

➤ **Always include protein.** Protein keeps you full and satisfied, builds lean muscle, and has very little impact on blood glucose. Aim for 3–4 ounces (about the size of your palm) of protein at each meal.

➤ **Include healthy fats at each meal.** Healthy fats keep you satisfied, help decrease hunger, and slow the absorption of glucose in your bloodstream.

➤ **Know your portion sizes.** We often don't realize that we overeat because we don't know what a portion size looks like. Become familiar with common portion sizes to be sure you are eating carbohydrates, protein, and fats in the right amounts.

Healthy Snacks

Eating well-balanced snacks can help stabilize blood glucose levels between meals. These snacks can help prevent mindless eating that sometimes happens when we get so hungry that we scarf down a sleeve of cookies instead of preparing a healthy meal. Be mindful of your portions—it's easy for a snack to grow into a meal. Below you will find a sample list of zero- and low-carbohydrate snacks. But note, although these are all low- to no-carbohydrate snacks, they do contain varying amounts of calories.

- ➤ 1 ounce string cheese or other cheese

- ➤ 1/4 cup nuts or seeds

- ➤ Small piece of fruit (for example, an apple, orange, or pear)

- ➤ Hard-boiled egg

- ➤ Celery with 1–2 tablespoons no-added-sugar nut butter or cream cheese

- ➤ 1/2 cup tuna or chicken salad

- ➤ Cottage cheese

- ➤ 1 slice of lean lunchmeat (for example, turkey or ham) rolled around a 1-ounce string cheese

- ➤ Raw vegetables with 1 tablespoon hummus

- ➤ Steamed vegetables (except for starch-heavy veggies like peas, corn, beans, potatoes, and sweet potatoes)

- ➤ 1/4 avocado with salsa

- ➤ 2 tablespoons pumpkin seeds

- ➤ 3 ounces leftover chicken breast or salmon

➤ 5–6 olives (green or black)*

➤ 1 large dill pickle*

➤ 1 serving of beef or turkey jerky*

➤ Cucumber or tomato slices with lemon and hot sauce

➤ Green salad without croutons or beans

➤ Sugar-free gelatin or sugar-free popsicle (check labels to find one with less than 5 grams of carbohydrates)

*May have high sodium content.

Healthy Swaps

Finding ways to make healthy swaps throughout the day and the week can really add up and have a positive impact on your overall diet. Here are some swaps to try. You'll be so surprised with some, you won't even miss the original!

Healthy Swaps

Instead of this . . .	Try this . . .
Sandwich bread	Wraps with hearty leafy greens (chard, kale, lettuce)
Mashed potatoes	Mashed cauliflower
Croutons	Walnuts
Mayonnaise	Mashed avocado
Pasta	Spaghetti squash
Sour cream	Plain Greek yogurt

Mindful Eating

In mindful eating, unlike in traditional "dieting," there are no good or bad foods. The idea is to be aware of which foods make you feel well and which make you feel unwell, either physically or emotionally.

Mindful eating is being fully immersed in the eating experience: you're smelling the food, feeling the texture while chewing, and focusing all of your senses on enjoying the experience. Where we can get into trouble is when we eat for pleasure without mindfulness. For example, you may sometimes eat more than you need if you are distracted by watching television or reading. This is called mindless eating.

Focusing on the sensation of eating and the feelings you have while eating can help you control cravings and overeating—controlling these two things can improve weight management, diabetes, blood pressure, and general health.

Tips for Mindful Eating

➤ Instead of eliminating foods, start by adding healthy foods that make you feel well. When you feel satisfied by nutritious foods, you might find yourself less likely to reach for less healthy foods.

➤ Listen to your body. Our bodies have ways to let us know that a food is good for us. For example, healthy foods often energize you, while unhealthy foods may make you feel sluggish.

➤ Use the scale below to help you figure out if you are hungry for a snack or a meal, or if you are eating for a reason other than hunger.

Hunger-Satiety Rating Scale

Full   10 = stuffed to the point of feeling sick

9 = very uncomfortably full, feel the need to loosen your belt

8 = uncomfortably full, feel stuffed

7 = very full, feel as if you have overeaten

6 = comfortably full, satisfied

Neutral   5 = comfortable, neither hungry nor full
               4 = beginning signs and symptoms of hunger
               3 = hungry with several hunger symptoms,
                   ready to eat
               2 = very hungry, unable to concentrate
Hungry   1 = starving, dizzy, irritable

Questions to Ask Yourself to Avoid Mindless Eating:

➤ Am I eating because I'm bored/nervous/upset or for some other reason that is not hunger?

➤ Do I ever get so busy that I don't know I'm hungry until I'm starving and have a headache—and then I overeat or choose unhealthy foods?

➤ Do I clean my plate even when I get full before my plate is empty? If your answer is "yes," use a smaller plate. Try to use a plate that is about 9 inches across. For reference, a dollar bill is just over 6 inches long.

Food and Emotions

Now that we've addressed general nutrition and healthy meal planning, let's switch back to looking at how food and emotions can affect life with diabetes and relationships (both with food and people). To start, let's debunk some of the common diabetes food myths and then look at things you can do to support a healthy attitude toward food.

Food Facts and Fictions

Sugar causes diabetes. **False**

The cause of diabetes varies depending on whether we are discussing type 1 or type 2 diabetes. In both cases, diabetes is *not* caused by sugar (unless a huge bag of sugar fell on you and somehow the only damage was that it crushed your pancreas). Details on what diabetes is and how you get diabetes are covered in Chapter 3.

People with diabetes can't eat sugar. **False**

Converting sugar to energy that our bodies can use requires insulin. For people with diabetes who either produce no insulin or insufficient amounts on their own, we compensate by taking insulin or medications or by doing things that improve our sensitivity to insulin.

You can reverse diabetes if you eat certain foods. **True *and* False**

There is confusion about the role food plays in diabetes. For a person with type 1 diabetes, there is no diet that will cure or reverse diabetes. Period. Some foods have a smaller impact on blood glucose than others and as a result require less insulin, but this still doesn't remove the need to take insulin. As you read earlier in Chapter 3, the body needs insulin even when not eating.

For people with type 2 diabetes, the topic is a bit less clear. The body's ability to produce insulin at diagnosis and beyond varies greatly from person to person. Type 2 diabetes progresses over time; this is why some people with type 2 diabetes who initially weren't required to take insulin, later may need it as their own insulin production decreases and/or their insulin resistance increases.

What does this have to do with our food fact/fiction? This is where some of the confusion rests. Lifestyle choices (healthy eating, exercise, and stress management) ***have*** been proven to be effective in helping to manage blood glucose levels and slowing the progression of type 2 diabetes. And for those who still produce a considerable amount of their own insulin, lifestyle changes may allow them to manage their diabetes without taking medication.

Diabetes is diagnosed when the concentration of glucose in the bloodstream exceeds a certain threshold (as measured in a series of glucose tests); therefore, some see being able to reduce blood glucose levels without medications to levels below the diagnostic threshold as having reversed diabetes. But to be clear, to date, the only proven way to get this type of reduction in blood glucose is through a healthy diet and regular exercise. There is no proven "miracle cure" for type 1 or type 2 diabetes that comes in the form of a single food, supplement, or drug.

People with diabetes have to give a great deal of thought to food and food choices. **True**

Food is a major component of diabetes management. Food choices and quantity have a direct and immediate impact on blood glucose levels, insulin requirements, and how we feel. Even when making healthy food choices, people with diabetes still have to think about how much carbohydrates they are eating, the overall composition of the meal, the timing of their food in relation to insulin and other medications, what kind of activity is about to take place, and, in many cases, the caloric content of the food.

Consider for a moment how much thinking a person who takes mealtime insulin is required to do before eating a simple meal:

➤ Check your blood glucose.

➤ Count the carbs in the meal.

➤ Determine the insulin dose to cover the carbs.

➤ Determine the insulin dose to "correct" the blood glucose before eating.

➤ Adjust the dose based on insulin-on-board and physical activity.

➤ Administer insulin via injection or a pump.

Let's look at the link between food and emotional wellness to help highlight strategies that foster a healthy relationship with food.

Building Blocks for Emotional Health and Healthy Eating

➤ **A sense of empowerment:** Understand how the body responds to different types of foods so that informed choices about what to buy and eat can be made. For example, Gary's blood glucose rises much more than expected when he eats bagels, while Diane's son Jackson experiences this kind of blood glucose response when he eats frozen yogurt. In these two cases, swapping whole-grain English muffins for bagels and real ice cream for frozen yogurt would give them both a similar food experience without the extreme spike in blood glucose. Knowledge is power and creates options.

➤ **A sense of belonging:** Share beliefs with family and friends about what healthy eating looks like, how special occasions are handled, and what words/tone are used to discuss food choices. You can create a sense of inclusion rather than directly or indirectly creating a separate set of eating rules/beliefs for your loved one with diabetes.

➤ **A sense of feeling supported:** Family and friends need to understand the work that goes into fitting diabetes into daily routines and special occasions. A simple thing like everyone starting the meal at the same time (after blood glucose check and medications are done) is a powerful message of support.

➤ **Freedom from judgment and shame:** Make sure your family/social circle understands that diabetes management isn't perfect. This applies to food choices as well as blood glucose levels.

In our culture, as in most cultures, food is central to celebrations, spending time together, entertaining, community events, and comfort. When attitudes toward food make people feel like they aren't (or shouldn't be) part of that culture, it creates feelings of isolation and being "different." Additionally, it's important to remember that diabetes doesn't take place in a vacuum. People with diabetes don't get a pass on other life challenges and struggles or the emotional impact of these life complexities. The combined effect of living with diabetes and the broader emotional struggles can lead to unhealthy eating patterns: binging, purging, sneaking, hoarding, and deprivation. We discussed these specific patterns in more detail in Chapter 3.

Warning: Food Traps Ahead

Diabetic Foods

One of our personal pet peeves is when you're at a grocery store and they have a section labeled *diabetic foods*. We can't help wondering what this means. Does the food have diabetes? Is there a new category on the food pyramid? Much like other labels used to describe foods, such as "low fat," "natural," or "lite," the term "diabetic food" is simply a marketing term, and these labeled foods don't provide any benefit for people living with diabetes.

FACTOID #13

There is no such thing, nor should there be such a thing, as a "diabetic food."

Some people may suggest that a food labeled "diabetic food" is sugar-free, low in carbohydrates, or low in fat. The truth is that many of the foods marketed as diabetic foods are highly processed and packed with artificial ingredients and chemicals and raise questions and concern about the potential negative impact on everyone's health, including people with diabetes.

The good news is, no special food or diet is required for people with diabetes. In most cases, what is healthy, well-balanced, and nutritious for people without diabetes is also appropriate for people with diabetes. The only exception would be when special consideration needs to be given for food allergies, celiac disease, or other specific food sensitivities/medical conditions.

Compared to a person with diabetes, a person without diabetes responds in similar ways to diets high in calories, trans fats, sodium, processed foods, and sugar. The only difference is that a person without diabetes produces enough insulin to keep the blood glucose within normal limits. However, both groups are subject to a host of other problems that come from a poor diet, such as weight gain, high cholesterol, high blood pressure, and so on. And don't forget about the insulin resistance that can develop or become worse. This increase in insulin resistance applies to people with or without diabetes, including individuals who have type 1 diabetes. A person living with type 1 diabetes can also develop type 2 diabetes.

Households across the country have struggled with questions like: "What should a person with diabetes eat?" "Do we have to cook two separate meals?" "Should I keep a collection of diabetic foods?" It is liberating and great news that healthy eating is essentially the same for all!

Food has components (calories, fat, protein, carbohydrates, vitamins, and minerals) and properties that determine how it is metabolized by the body (used for energy, stored as fat, and passed as waste). How much you need of each type of nutrient is based on your unique requirements, body type, size, and activity level, not on whether or not you have diabetes. In most cases, diets that contain lots of whole foods (fruits, vegetables, nuts, seeds, whole grains), lean sources of protein, and healthy fats (olives, coconut, avocado, nuts) and are consumed in appropriate portions, support the body's ability to maintain a healthy weight, stabilize blood glucose, and fight illness and disease.

FACTOID #14

> Foods that are best for people with diabetes are basically the same as what is healthy for people without diabetes.

Forbidden Foods

Now that you know there is no such thing as "diabetic foods," you can probably guess what we're going to say about forbidden foods. Yup—there's no such thing. Unless your loved one with diabetes has food allergies or celiac disease (gluten intolerance), there aren't any foods that are forbidden specifically because a person has diabetes.

"Kryptonite" Food

Although there is no such thing as forbidden food, many people with diabetes, especially those with type 1 diabetes, have certain foods that act like "kryptonite" for them. (Kryptonite was the substance that even the comic book hero, Superman, couldn't handle. Exposure to it took his superpowers away.) Kryptonite foods make blood glucose levels skyrocket inexplicably and stay high for hours, no matter what the person with diabetes does with insulin dosing or exercise to try to control it.

FACTOID #15

> Bagels are Gary's kryptonite food. Soft pretzels take a full 24 hours to work their way out of Diane's son Jackson's system.

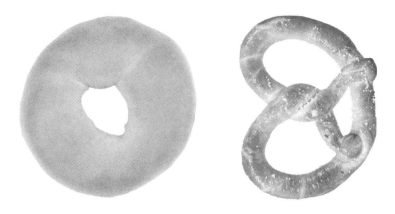

"Kryptonite" foods can vary from person to person, but some common offenders include pizza, Chinese food, soft pretzels, and frozen yogurt. Knowledge is power. If people with diabetes know their "kryptonite foods," they can decide whether they want to endure the blood glucose rollercoaster that will likely follow if these foods are eaten. Your loved one should know that "strange" blood glucose levels are not his or her fault. It's just part of living with a complex and sometimes unpredictable condition.

I'm Eating It, but Should You?
Rules and Attitudes Pertaining to Food

Related to our thoughts about food choices are our beliefs about how people with diabetes "should" eat. Even when we accept that healthy food is the same for all of us, there are often expectations that people with diabetes should automatically acquire some superhuman willpower when it comes to temptation, hectic schedules, convenience, and cravings. Most of these attitudes come from good intentions, but they can make people with diabetes feel judged and shamed.

SECRET STRATEGY #7

Watch out for trap phrases like, "Are you allowed to eat that? Doesn't that raise your blood glucose?"

Few of us can say that we make healthy choices 100% of the time. And even if *you* have made that commitment to your eating habits, it was likely a decision that you made based on your life situation, your priorities, your goals, and your ability to fulfill those goals. Here are ways that you can support healthy eating in your household and help your loved one with diabetes:

> ➤ Make healthy options available at group gatherings

> ➤ Model healthy food choices yourself

> ➤ Rid your pantry and fridge of processed and packaged foods

> ➤ Have celebrations centered around activities in addition to or rather than food

> ➤ Share favorite healthy recipes that you've tried and like

For a number of psychosocial reasons, people have a powerful desire to fit in with friends and family. Sharing a common practice of clean or clean**er** eating (eating whole foods that are minimally processed) in social settings makes it much easier for everyone to maintain healthy eating habits and have a sense of belonging.

Making statements and asking frequent questions about food choices typically has the reverse effect and fosters resentment and tension. When there is one set of food beliefs or practices for people with diabetes and separate practices for everyone else, this can leave people with diabetes feeling as if they aren't "normal."

There's little ability to influence what and how others outside your family eat, so providing a sense of togetherness at home is a powerful way to help offset exclusionary feelings that happen in other environments. As a person living with a loved one with diabetes, you can play a big part in creating a *"no place like home"* feeling.

Ways to Create a Sense of Togetherness

➤ Create mealtime routines that allow time for diabetes tasks, such as checking blood glucose and taking medications.

➤ Use shared terminology when referring to food choices, for example, "strong food" and "weak food," or "real food" and "party food," not "your food" and "our food."

➤ Have the same food choices for everybody. Don't use "diabetes food" or statements that suggest a person can't eat something that others are eating because of diabetes.

SECRET STRATEGY #8

Rather than making frequent comments (or asking questions) about your loved one's food choices, model healthy eating patterns yourself and make good choices readily available.

Don't Be the "Food Police"

You realize that food choices affect blood glucose and you worry about your loved one with diabetes. This concern may lead to frequent questions about what they ate, when they ate, why they ate, or if they ate . . . which quickly adds up to a never-ending food interrogation. Resist the urge to become the "food police" and instead refer back to Chapter 4 to see other ways to communicate about food and diabetes without policing.

Food Do's and Don'ts

Food Do's

➤ Do make healthy food choices available for the whole family.

➤ Do look for celebration activities that aren't centered on food.

➤ Do try to swap healthy choices for unhealthy ones in your pantry/fridge.

➤ Do realize that nobody is going to make healthy food choices all the time, and that's OK.

➤ Do create premeal schedules/practices that allow time for diabetes tasks.

Food Don'ts

➤ Don't keep a separate "diabetic" food shelf. (An exception would be a supply of items to treat low blood glucose.)

➤ Don't have different standards/eating practices for people with diabetes versus yourself or others in the family. This is especially important between siblings.

➤ Don't assign yourself the role of "food police."

➤ Don't nag, badger, or otherwise browbeat your loved one with diabetes on issues related to food.

....

Dining Out

Dining out creates challenges for anyone trying to eat healthy and watch their weight. Portions are typically much larger than a standard serving size and contain tons of sodium. Sauces can be loaded with hidden sugar and fat, and nutrition information like calories and carbs is rarely listed. Not knowing what is in the foods makes it difficult to make healthy choices. And it is almost impossible to make correct insulin dosing decisions.

Frequent dining out often contributes to weight gain and a host of health concerns including cardiovascular disease, high cholesterol, and high blood pressure. And while restaurants offering healthy, clean food are gaining popularity, these dining options can be very expensive and hard to find.

Top Restaurant Survival Tips
(for Everyone!)

➤ Ask the server how things are prepared. Look for grilled or baked rather than fried or sautéed foods.

➤ Ask the server to hold or put sauces/dressings on the side.

➤ Split desserts or large servings with your partner or others at your table, or put half in a take-home container as soon as the food arrives at the table.

➤ Many chain restaurants provide nutrition information on their websites. Look them up on your computer or cell phone and make your choices before you go. This step helps you avoid being tempted by less healthy options (which is really easy when you're hungry!).

➤ Enjoy a small snack containing protein and healthy fat (such as an apple with peanut butter) before dining out so hunger doesn't lead to overeating.

➤ Find one or two restaurants in the area that consistently offer healthy options and make these go-to choices for dining out or takeout.

➤ Avoid or limit daily alcohol (one drink or less for women and two drinks or less for men, according to the American Diabetes Association). One drink is equal to a 12-ounce beer, 5-ounce glass of wine, or 1.5 ounces of distilled spirits (vodka, whiskey, gin, etc.).

Alcohol and Diabetes

It is important to understand how alcohol affects blood glucose in people with diabetes. Even though many alcoholic drinks (including beer, sweet wine, and most mixed drinks) contain carbohydrates that raise blood glucose, alcohol can also cause blood glucose to drop several hours later. This pattern of high blood glucose followed by low blood glucose after drinking is dangerous.

The reason for the delayed drop in blood glucose is this: The liver stores glucose (sugar) and releases small amounts of it into the bloodstream throughout the day and night. The body counts on this steady release of glucose to provide energy for the brain and other vital organs. When alcohol is present, the liver essentially cuts back on the release of glucose so it can process the alcohol. This reduction in the liver's glucose production is what can cause hypoglycemia (low blood glucose), particularly if the person hasn't eaten and has taken his or her usual doses of insulin or medication.

Be Careful to Not Mistake Hypoglycemia for Drunkenness

Symptoms of drunkenness and hypoglycemia can be similar: sleepiness, dizziness, slurred speech, and disorientation. Not only do people with diabetes have difficulty recognizing their lows after drinking, but so do people around them. If you are with someone with diabetes who is exhibiting these symptoms, try to check blood glucose and do not assume he or she just needs to "sleep it off." When in doubt, assume that blood glucose is low and feed the person something containing at least 15 grams of carbohydrates, such as a regular (sugar-sweetened) beverage, and check blood glucose again in 20 minutes. Call 9-1-1 for immediate help if you are unable to get the person to eat or drink or if his or her symptoms do not improve.

Combining physical activity with alcohol can be particularly dangerous. For example, drinking beer right after a hard workout, or having mixed drinks while dancing at a club, greatly increases the risk of hypoglycemia. Alcohol is best avoided during periods of heightened physical activity. If alcohol and physical activity are combined, encourage the consumption of plenty of extra carbohydrates.

FACTOID #16

Because alcohol can lower blood glucose in a delayed manner, it is important to take precautions to avoid serious hypoglycemia after drinking.

For a host of reasons, the buddy system is important for everyone to adopt when drinking alcohol. Having a buddy who understands how alcohol can affect blood glucose levels is invaluable to a person with diabetes.

Practices to Sip By

➤ Encourage your partner to check blood glucose before drinking alcohol and more frequently after drinking, for up to 24 hours, including during the night. Set an alarm!

➤ Check blood glucose before going to bed to make sure it is at a safe level. Generally, a blood glucose below 100 mg/dL will require a carbohydrate-containing snack.

➤ Encourage snacking on small amounts of carbohydrate at hourly intervals when drinking alcohol.

➤ Those who take insulin or medications that stimulate the pancreas to produce more insulin should ask their health care team about reducing their doses overnight after drinking.

KEY POINTS

➤ Food has concrete properties that are true for everyone. There is no such thing as a "diabetic food."

➤ Food plays a big role in our culture and relationships and therefore in our emotional health. Try to create a sense of belonging related to food.

➤ Simple meal-planning strategies make healthy eating easier for everyone.

➤ Beware: have you become the "food police"?

➤ Paying attention to preparation method, portion size, and frequency of eating out can make dining out healthier.

➤ Drinking alcohol can cause low blood glucose in a person with diabetes for up to 24 hours after drinking. Extra blood glucose checks and combining food with alcohol will reduce the risks.

➤ Symptoms of drunkenness and hypoglycemia (low blood glucose) are similar.

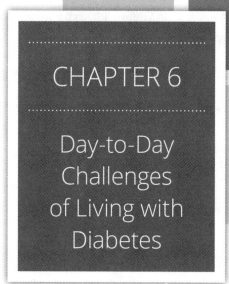

CHAPTER 6

Day-to-Day Challenges of Living with Diabetes

*I*nsanity is often defined as doing the same thing over and over again and expecting different results. Unfortunately, this is what we see all the time when people are attempting to manage their blood glucose levels. There comes a time (lots of times, actually) in everyone's life with diabetes when changes are needed. What worked well a few months (or even a few weeks) ago may not work today. Over time, bodies change and treatments need to be adjusted as well.

Pattern Management

There's a big difference between an occasional unexpected high or low blood glucose level and a *pattern* of out-of-range readings. "Pattern management" is the process used to identify trends and make adjustments to various parts of a diabetes management plan to help bring blood glucose levels into target range. This step requires a good system for collecting and analyzing data and an even better system for making adjustments based on what the data teach us.

SECRET STRATEGY #9

Log your readings! People who record their blood glucose values have better control than those who don't.

In supporting a loved one with diabetes, you can certainly assist with recordkeeping and the analysis of data. In some ways, your objectivity may even make it easier to spot potential problem areas. Recordkeeping keeps everyone involved and accountable. It also lets you see what's working and what isn't. In addition to written logs (using logbooks or log sheets), blood glucose data can be collected by downloading meters and printing out a report. Meters such as the Livongo meter automatically collect and store blood glucose information through wireless technology. There are also smartphone apps that allow for simple data tracking. Popular logging apps include MySugr, Glooko, Dario, and Glucose Buddy.

Blood glucose analysis can get fairly involved and should be done with the help of an experienced diabetes health professional. It is important to make sure that the health care team has the right information. To perform a good analysis, it is helpful to start with at least a few weeks' worth of blood glucose data. If you're not using software to capture data, using columns for different times of the day helps detect patterns. For example, put all of the pre-breakfast readings in one column, pre-lunch in another, and so on. Adding in a blood glucose check 2 hours after a meal is started is also helpful to evaluate how high blood glucose levels are "spiking" after certain meals or types of foods.

When evaluating data, check each phase of the day individually. If your loved one is experiencing multiple lows at the same time of day, an adjustment is probably in order. Likewise, if a significant number of readings are above-target at the same time of day, an adjustment may be needed.

Patterns to look for and discuss with your health care team:

➤ Frequent low blood glucose levels

➤ Frequent morning high blood glucose levels

➤ Frequent high or low blood glucose levels that happen at the same time of day

➤ Timing of food, medication, activity, and any illness

Going over this information with your health care provider is the best way to make informed adjustments to a plan. For example, here are 2 weeks of data for March. Nora takes multiple daily insulin injections, and her target blood glucose range is 70–160 mg/dL before meals and below 200 mg/dL after meals.

Blood Glucose Data Collected Over 2 Weeks

	Before Break-fast	After Break-fast	Before Lunch	After Lunch	Before Dinner	After Dinner	At Bed-time
Monday 3/1	95	166	74		127		98
Tuesday 3/2	175		87	144	131		135
Wednesday 3/3	199		63		77	298	149
Thursday 3/4	99	190	58		83		103
Friday 3/5	215		80	133	116		99
Saturday 3/6	116		117		100	202	117
Sunday 3/7	81	175	204		64		82

(continues)

Blood Glucose Data Collected Over 2 Weeks (*Continued*)

	Before Break-fast	After Break-fast	Before Lunch	After Lunch	Before Dinner	After Dinner	At Bed-time
Monday 3/8	148		65	162	95		110
Tuesday 3/9	216		110		266	281	199
Wednesday 3/10	189		57		103		133
Thursday 3/11	130	158	44		87		82
Friday 3/12	255		98	183	88		116
Saturday 3/13	118		111		118	311	207
Sunday 3/14	205		59		89		120

Do you notice any patterns? Tally up how often Nora is below, within, and above target.

How Often Were Values Below, Within, or Above Target?

	Before Breakfast	Before Lunch	Before Dinner	At Bedtime
Below target	0	6	1	0
Within target	7	7	12	12
Above target	7	1	1	2

Nora is having a lot of above-target blood glucose readings before breakfast and a number of below-target readings before lunch. There is also a pattern of above-target readings soon after dinner. Patterns can also be detected by looking at data from a continuous glucose monitor (CGM) download.

Here is a report for a patient named Ben, an 8-year-old boy with type 1 diabetes who uses an insulin pump. This "modal day" report for Ben reveals a pattern of low blood

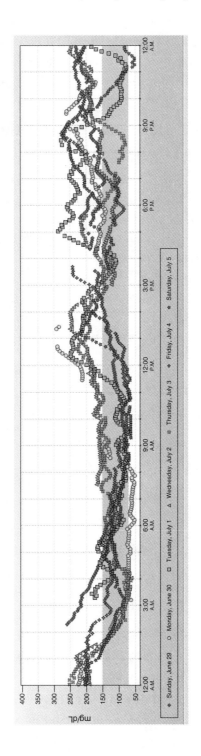

glucose values in the morning hours, followed by some temporarily elevated blood glucose values after dinner and a gradual rise in the evening.

Be a Blood Glucose Detective

You've successfully completed the most important part of pattern management: detecting the problem areas. Now comes the fun part: finding the optimal solution. Put on your detective cap. You will need to consider the possible "suspects," investigate, and narrow it down to solve the case. And don't forget to call on the expertise of your health care team to find the best possible answer.

The "usual suspects" can vary from case to case. There are so many factors that influence blood glucose levels. Some of the following scenarios could be causing out-of-range blood glucose levels:

➤ Too much or too little food

➤ Unusual foods, such as restaurant meals

➤ Improper insulin dosing formulas

➤ Errors in calculating carbs or insulin doses

➤ A need to add/switch medications or change a dosage

➤ Pump infusion set changes

➤ Day-to-day variations in physical activity (including exercise and daily chores)

➤ Stressful or emotional situations

➤ Illness or infection

It is also helpful to see if lows tend to follow highs, highs tend to follow lows, or highs tend to stay high (or lows tend to stay low), since these types of patterns can reveal the source of consecutive out-of-range readings.

When it comes to solving the mystery, the culprit is not always one of the "usual suspects." As an example, a curbside baggage handler at the airport discovered that his daytime blood glucose was greatly influenced by how much luggage he processed. On the busiest travel days (Fridays and Sundays), his blood glucose levels were much lower than the rest of the week. A simple reduction to his mealtime insulin on busy days solved the problem.

Once you've pinpointed the likely suspect, devising a practical solution is often obvious. If you're having difficulty interpreting your loved one's data or coming up with a solution, or you just want an expert to verify that your conclusions are sound, ask your physician or diabetes educator for assistance.

Even if your A1C is satisfactory, it is worthwhile to review blood glucose data once or twice a month. Remember, an A1C only reflects an average blood glucose: you could be experiencing patterns of highs and lows that "average out" somewhere in the middle. It is equally (if not more) important that the day-to-day blood glucose levels are within your target range as often as possible.

POP QUIZ

The "gold standard" for evaluating blood glucose control is:

A. A1C

B. The number of times the blood glucose is low

C. The amount of time spent within your target range

ANSWER: **C, with a little A and B.** A1C correlates with the risk of long-term complications, and hypoglycemia is certainly something we strive to avoid. But ultimately, the amount of time we spend within our target range translates into the best combination of safety, performance, and quality of life.

Sexual Intimacy

Remember those topics that made you blush and giggle when you were in health class in school? It's time for a reunion! None of us are completely immune to embarrassing topics or feeling awkward when it comes to talking about our body, sex, and intimacy. It happens to everyone. As clinical diabetes educators, we deal with body parts and body functions all day long. But nobody embraces the concept of addressing highly personal topics around strangers. One of the beautiful things about books is being able to address topics like intimacy without anyone seeing you blush.

Diabetes can play a role in sex and intimacy. Getting up to speed in this area will help you know what to expect and make it easier to have open conversations with your loved one and health care providers. Diabetes can contribute to erectile dysfunction, loss of sex drive, vaginal dryness, pain during intercourse, and hypoglycemia during foreplay and intercourse. Many people without diabetes experience these challenges (except for hypoglycemia), so if they have become part of your life, you are definitely not alone.

FACTOID #17

Erectile dysfunction (impotency) is one of the most common complications of both type 1 and type 2 diabetes.

In most cases, there are effective treatment options. Your health care provider can help you determine which will work best for you and your partner. The key is recognizing that sexual health is part of overall diabetes management and needs to be discussed openly with a health care provider.

How and when to bring this up should be mutually agreed upon by you and your partner with diabetes. If you recognize issues related to intimacy, ask (don't tell) your partner that you would like to address it with the doctor. If he or she doesn't feel comfortable bringing it up, ask if you can discuss it with the doctor, either as a couple or by yourself.

Hypoglycemia can also come into play where sexual activity is concerned. Pay attention to the "activity" part of that phrase. Sexual activity burns energy and raises your heart rate. So the rules for managing blood glucose during sexual activity are the same as the rules for other forms of exercise. Make sure blood glucose is in a safe range before engaging, have a snack first (if necessary), and watch for delayed lows after extended periods of sexual activity.

SECRET STRATEGY #10

If your partner uses a "tubed" insulin pump, learn how to "disconnect" the tubes when the mood arises if he or she prefers to remove the pump. And give a gentle reminder to *reconnect* afterwards!

Body Image

Body image can also affect our comfort level with intimacy. Issues related to body image plague us all. Society spends a great deal of time and money telling us how tall, curvy, muscular, tan, tight, and smooth our bodies *should* be. This constant barrage of messages from all forms of mass media and social media can make anybody feel like they don't measure up.

People with diabetes may also be self-conscious about the medical devices they use or wear. Some are hesitant to show their insulin pump, infusion set, or CGM site, while others are uncomfortable about having others watch them check blood glucose or give injections. It is important that you let your partner know that these types of things do not make him or her less desirable to you.

Miss Idaho, Sierra Sandison, sent a powerful positive message when she wore an insulin pump in her bikini while walking the runway of a beauty contest. She chose to show the world that beauty comes with all types of accessories and packaging. This message is particularly important and critical for young women living with diabetes.

Your loved one might not be ready to "walk the runway" with all the diabetes paraphernalia, and that's OK. You can do your part by learning about the diabetes equipment and routines, and as mentioned above, telling your partner how much you care for him or her with, or without, all the diabetes stuff. For additional information about intimacy, read *Sex and Diabetes: For Him and For Her* by Janis Roszler and Donna Rice (American Diabetes Association).

Traveling with Diabetes

Travel can present special challenges for people with diabetes. Because of changes in meals, activity, and schedules, blood glucose levels may vary more than usual when a person with diabetes is away from home. Nobody wants diabetes to get in the way of having a fun (or productive) time, so here are some travel tips to share with your loved one with diabetes.

Travel Tip #1: Double Pack

Nothing will wreak havoc on a trip more than losing or running out of (or forgetting) key supplies. Think like Santa:

Make a list, and check it twice. Include everything you need on a daily or occasional basis to manage your diabetes. Bring everything from insulin/medication to monitoring supplies to hypoglycemia treatments to batteries for your equipment. And then when packing, make a *second* set of everything. This will cover you just in case the first set is lost, stolen, damaged, or confiscated. When you travel, ask your partner to hold on to a complete backup set of diabetes supplies, just in case.

SECRET STRATEGY #11

Bring a backup set of supplies for your partner/loved one when you travel together. Include equipment, medications, and disposable items.

Travel Tip #2: Get Ready for Time-Zone Changes

Multiple time zone changes (going and returning) can have a huge impact on blood glucose control, particularly for people who take insulin. In most cases, individuals who take insulin will need to alter the timing and doses of long-acting (basal) insulin to prevent gaps and overlaps in insulin coverage. It is generally a good idea to take long-acting (basal) insulin doses according to your *home* clock. For example, if your loved one normally takes basal insulin at 8:00 P.M. and you travel west across two time zones, taking it at 6:00 P.M. at your destination would keep the doses 24 hours apart. If you travel east across two time zones, taking it at 10:00 P.M. at your destination would keep the doses 24 hours apart. Ask your loved one's health care provider for suggestions before your trip.

Pump users have it much easier. Simply update the clock in the pump to match the local time upon arrival at your destination, and the pump's basal insulin delivery should match up nicely to your new sleep cycle.

SECRET STRATEGY #12

Remind your loved one to update the time in his or her pump, meter, and CGM to match the local time when you arrive.

Travel Tip #3: Prepare to Be Screened

Airport screening procedures vary from country to country. In the U.S., no more than 3 ounces of gels and liquids are allowed through security checkpoints, so make sure your loved one's hypoglycemia treatments are in "solid" form. Although manufacturers of pumps, meters, and continuous monitors sometimes warn against exposing devices to x-ray equipment, there is no evidence that diabetes equipment/supplies are damaged by airport screening machines. If your loved one wears a device that triggers an alert when passing through screening machines, let the security personnel know that you wear (or carry) a device for your diabetes. Typically, security officials will simply check your hands for traces of explosive materials and then send you on your way.

Travel Tip #4: Maintain Your Physical Activity

When traveling, many people with diabetes let their normal workout program slide. Decreasing normal activity can cause a loss of insulin sensitivity, resulting in higher-than-usual blood glucose levels. "Transit" days, in particular, may involve long periods of sitting in one position. Ask your loved one's health care provider about the possibility of increasing the usual insulin/medication doses for these situations. Or better yet, do what you can to maintain consistent workouts while traveling. The type of workout may be different than usual, but any form of exercise is better than none at all.

Make use of hotel fitness centers, walk/jog/bike to explore your new surroundings, or bring along your own workout videos or other exercise equipment. If you belong to a health club at home, see if the club has a branch that you can access near where you'll be staying.

Travel Tip #5: Protect Your Insulin

Insulin is stable at room temperature for up to 1 month. There is not usually a need to refrigerate insulin while traveling. However, if the temperature at your destination is in excess of 90 degrees Fahrenheit (32 degrees Celsius) and your accommodations are not air-conditioned, either keep the insulin in a refrigerator or bring along a temperature-controlled case for your insulin vials and pens. If you use a pump and expose it to high temperatures (on a beach or while sightseeing), consider changing the insulin in the pump and tubing on a more frequent basis.

Travel Tip #6: Be Emergency-Ready

Be sure to bring hypoglycemia treatments and a glucagon kit with you when traveling, and keep them with you at all times. Because food, activity, and schedules may be radically different than when at home, the chances of severe low blood glucose levels are much greater when traveling. It is also a good idea to bring along a first aid kit for handling minor illnesses and injuries.

SECRET STRATEGY #13

If your partner takes insulin, always have hypoglycemia treatments, including a glucagon kit, in *your* possession when traveling.

Dealing with Sick Days

There are only a handful of situations in which people with diabetes may be unable to fend for themselves. Sick days are one of them. A person's ability to make rational decisions and perform routine diabetes management tasks can be compromised when he or she is ill. The support of a loved one or caregiver can make a tremendous difference on sick days.

Sick days include more than just routine colds and the flu. Any situation that places a major stress on the body can prompt a sick day. These situations may include:

> ➤ Developing an infection (of the skin, toe/foot, vaginal area, urinary tract, gastrointestinal tract, respiratory tract, or gums)

> ➤ Developing a fever (which is usually a symptom of an infection)

> ➤ Undergoing surgery (from minor outpatient procedures to major surgery)

> ➤ Undergoing treatments for other health problems (such as radiation or chemotherapy)

> ➤ Having a serious injury (bone breaks, muscle tears/ pulls, tendon/ligament damage)

> ➤ Having significant nausea (possibly involving diarrhea, vomiting, or inability to eat/drink)

Infections, unfortunately, are more common in people with diabetes, mostly when blood glucose levels are elevated. Infection-fighting white blood cells do not work well when blood glucose is high. Extra glucose in the bloodstream also provides nourishment for viruses and bacteria. All of the "sick day" situations listed above cause the body to produce stress hormones, which drive the blood glucose levels even higher and make insulin less effective. In fact, illness and uncontrolled diabetes actually feed on one another. Illness makes blood glucose higher, and higher blood glucose levels make it harder to recover from illness.

Ketones may be elevated during an illness, particularly in people with type 1 diabetes (ketones are far less common in people with type 2 diabetes). Ketones are acids that accumulate when sugar (glucose) is unavailable to be burned for energy, as is the case when the body is severely insulin resistant because of an illness/infection. The buildup of ketones is called **ketosis**. When ketosis becomes excessive and is combined with dehydration, a life-threatening condition known as **diabetic ketoacidosis (DKA)** may develop. During DKA, the blood becomes so acidic that severe body aches and vomiting often occur. Breathing can become very deep and labored, and the breath may take on a "spoiled fruit" smell as the lungs attempt to rid the body of acid through exhalation. Treatment for DKA requires an immediate trip to the nearest emergency room. Left untreated, DKA can lead to permanent brain damage or death.

Caregiver's Role on Sick Days

As indicated above, it is challenging, yet important, to manage blood glucose levels during sick days. Even if your loved one is not eating as much as usual, he or she needs to continue taking diabetes medication and basal/long-acting insulin. Without basal insulin, the blood glucose can go dangerously high and ketosis/ketoacidosis may develop.

It is important to check blood glucose on a regular basis on sick days, so make sure you know how to use the meter. Ketones may also need to be checked (particularly in people with type 1 diabetes). Be prepared with either urine Ketostix or a blood glucose meter that can also measure ketones in a blood sample (Precision Xtra or NovaMax Plus). If blood glucose is unusually high or ketones are present, communicate this information to your loved one's health care provider. The health care provider may recommend extra basal insulin on sick days. The basal insulin increase is used in addition to correction bolus doses to get, and keep, blood glucose levels in a healthy range.

Keep in mind that insulin will not absorb properly into the bloodstream in someone who is not adequately hydrated. It is essential for people with diabetes to drink plenty of fluids on sick days—preferably clear, caffeine-free fluids. Most adults should consume about 1 cup per hour while awake; small children should consume about 1/2 cup per hour. Calories (in the form of easily digestible carbohydrates and a modest amount of protein) are also needed on sick days to provide a source of energy. Good choices include bread/crackers, cereal, soup, soft fruit, rice, eggs, and small portions of cheese, peanut butter, and lean meats.

Some over-the-counter medications for things like colds, congestion, headaches, and nausea warn against use by people with diabetes. In most cases, this is because the medication contains sugar or some other substance that can raise blood glucose a small amount. It is not usually a problem to take these medications as long as attention is paid to blood glucose levels. If in doubt, check with your health care team. Also, be aware that medications that contain acetaminophen (the pain reliever/anti-inflammatory found in Tylenol products and many other over-the-counter medications) can artificially raise glucose values on CGMs. If you must take acetaminophen (or take it accidentally), it is best to ignore the CGM for the next several hours and perform routine fingersticks instead.

Here is a quick sick-day toolkit for caregivers of people with diabetes:

➤ Know how to use your loved one's meter.

➤ Continue to administer basal doses of insulin.

➤ Check ketones daily.

➤ Push lots of fluids.

➤ Provide easily digested carbs.

In the event a mild illness takes a turn for the worse, contact your health care team and/or go to a local hospital's emergency department immediately. Be on the lookout for any of these symptoms:

➤ Repeated bouts of vomiting

➤ Prolonged diarrhea

➤ Large/high ketone levels

➤ Very high blood glucose levels that do not respond to the usual treatments

➤ High fever that does not respond to fever-reducing medication

➤ Erratic behaviors (delirium)

Physical Activity

Throughout this book, the topic of physical activity has popped up multiple times. Other than insulin (and other diabetes medications), physical activity is the primary tool we have for reducing blood glucose levels. It does this in three ways: *1*) by making our muscles more sensitive to insulin, *2*) by contributing to weight loss (which also improves insulin sensitivity), and *3*) by burning glucose directly for energy. Physical activity also plays a key role in preventing or reversing many of the serious health problems that diabetes can cause. It improves blood flow/circulation to the brain, heart, legs, feet, and vital organs. It helps to reduce blood pressure and cholesterol levels. It improves mood and helps us to fight stress. And it is a good way to maintain flexibility and full range of motion. In many ways, physical activity is like a very powerful medication for the challenges faced by people with diabetes every day.

As a support person, there are many things you can do on behalf of your loved one, but physical activity is not one of them. Here are ways that you can encourage and enable an active lifestyle for your loved one with diabetes:

1. Be active yourself. People are more likely to be active when surrounded by other active people.

2. Pair up. Invite the person with diabetes to join you in active pursuits such as walking, gardening, dancing, cycling, and sports.

3. Provide access to exercise equipment (or classes) by joining a health club or purchasing something to use at home.

4. Help open up your loved one's schedule so that he or she has time for scheduled activity.

5. Resist the urge to nag. Often, nagging will produce the opposite of the desired effect.

6. Ask your partner's diabetes team to help you develop blood glucose management strategies for exercise. This is particularly important for individuals who take insulin to prevent hypoglycemia. It is often necessary to reduce mealtime (rapid-acting) insulin when exercise is going to take place after a meal. For premeal activity, extra carbohydrates may be needed to prevent hypoglycemia.

FACTOID #18

There are a lot of things you can do on your loved one's behalf, but exercise is *not* one of them.

KEY POINTS

➤ You, as a support person, are in a unique position to detect blood glucose patterns and pinpoint solutions.

➤ Sexual issues are common in people with diabetes. Open communication with your partner and his or her health care team is essential.

➤ With proper preparation, diabetes should not interfere with or restrict travel.

➤ Be prepared to assume some diabetes management responsibilities when your loved one is ill.

➤ Find ways to support your loved one in being physically active without being "pushy."

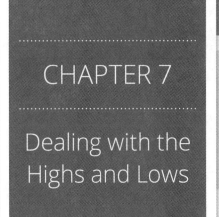

CHAPTER 7

Dealing with the Highs and Lows

Hypoglycemia (Low Blood Glucose)

Perhaps no other aspect of diabetes is more important to the support person than knowing how to deal with a loved one's low blood glucose reaction (hypoglycemia). While most people with diabetes prefer to take care of their own business when it comes to daily management, hypoglycemia is a major exception. In many instances, people with diabetes are unable to properly treat themselves when low blood glucose takes place. The more prepared and equipped you are to handle your loved one's hypoglycemia, the better.

Let's focus on the causes and all-important treatments for hypoglycemia. Low blood glucose is usually defined as a level of less than 70 mg/dL (3.9 mmol/L). In people without diabetes, this almost never happens because the pancreas only produces insulin on an as-needed basis and does so in just the right amounts. Low blood glucose can occur in people with diabetes who take insulin or medications that cause the body to produce more insulin (sulfonylureas and meglitinides). Any time there is slightly more insulin than is needed for a given situation, low blood glucose can occur. Examples include:

➤ Increased physical activity

➤ Multitasking

➤ Missed or delayed meals/snacks

➤ Overestimation of carbohydrates

➤ Taking the wrong insulin type

➤ Accidental overdosing of insulin

➤ Vomiting

➤ Alcohol consumption

Mild Low Glucose Levels

Virtually all systems of the body are affected by low blood glucose, but none quite as much as the brain. Brain cells are picky about their fuel source. These cells prefer to burn sugar for energy. When the blood glucose drops below 70 mg/dL or is dropping very quickly and heading low, the brain triggers a surge of adrenaline. Adrenaline, in turn, partially blocks the action of insulin and stimulates the liver to secrete glucose into the bloodstream. Adrenaline also causes a number of physical symptoms: rapid heartbeat, perspiration, shaking, hunger, and a generally anxious feeling. These are the same symptoms that occur when you are under intense stress, like when you're driving and the car in front of you suddenly slams on the brakes. When mild hypoglycemia occurs, most people with diabetes who are old enough to think for themselves are more than capable of consuming food or drink without assistance to raise their blood glucose level.

Moderate Low Glucose Levels

If blood glucose levels drop into the 50s or 40s (3–2 mmol/L), the brain begins losing the ability to function properly. Confusion usually sets in, accompanied by dizziness and weakness. Speech may become slurred. Unusual emotions such as irritability or despair can occur. Vision may become blurred. The person experiencing the low will usually have a difficult time thinking clearly and coordinating movements. The person may or may not be able to think rationally. However, your loved one will usually know that he or she needs to consume food to raise blood glucose and will still have the ability to eat or drink. At this point, a support person may need to fetch food or drink for treating the low.

Severe Low Glucose Levels

An extreme or prolonged low blood glucose reaction may cause loss of consciousness, seizure, or a loss of self-control such that the victim is unable to consciously eat or drink. Severe lows, by definition, require outside assistance and are usually treated with an injection of glucagon or an intravenous infusion of dextrose.

It is important to note that hypoglycemia does not always follow neat, tidy steps from mild to moderate to severe. Individuals who have had diabetes for many years and have experienced many episodes of hypoglycemia often develop something called "hypoglycemia unawareness." The brain loses the ability to detect mild hypoglycemia and does not generate the usual early warning signs such as shaking, sweating, and rapid heartbeat. The first indication that blood glucose is low may be confusion or profound behavior changes. So it is necessary to be prepared for handling hypoglycemia at any state—from mild to severe—by following the instructions below.

FACTOID #19

Hypoglycemia does not always progress nicely from mild to moderate to severe. Severe low glucose can occur with little to no warning.

Treating Low Glucose Levels

Diabetes can be sneaky. The symptoms of high and low blood glucose are sometimes hard to distinguish. If you suspect that a loved one is having a low and there is a glucose meter available, take a few seconds to check blood glucose levels. Getting an exact reading will also help to determine how much food will be needed to treat the low. Take the time to learn and practice doing blood glucose checks using your loved one's meter.

FACTOID #20

Learn how to do a blood glucose check using your loved one's meter *before* an emergency arises.

There is no one-size-fits-all treatment for hypoglycemia. Proper treatment depends on a person's body size and how low the blood glucose levels is. The bigger a person is and the lower the glucose level, the more carbs he or she will need. The table below provides a good starting point.

Suggested Carbohydrates Needed to Raise Blood Glucose to Approximately 120 mg/dL (6.7 mmol/L)

Weight	Blood Glucose				
	60s (3.3–3.9)	50s (2.8–3.2)	40s (2.2–2.7)	30s (1.7–2.1)	20s (1.1–1.6)
<60 lb (28 kg)	9 g	11 g	13 g	15 g	17 g
60–100 lb (29–47 kg)	11 g	13 g	15 g	17 g	19 g
101–160 lb (48–76 kg)	14 g	16 g	19 g	21 g	24 g
161–220 lb (77–105 kg)	18 g	22 g	25 g	28 g	32 g
>220 lb (>105 kg)	28 g	33 g	38 g	43 g	48 g

For example, someone who weighs 150 lb and has a blood glucose of 65 mg/dL will need approximately 14 grams of carbohydrate. Someone who weighs 210 lb and has a blood glucose of 48 mg/dL will require 25 grams.

For those who use a continuous glucose monitor (CGM), the **rate of change** can also be taken into account. If the blood glucose is low and dropping quickly, you may need to double the amount of carbohydrate (see example below).

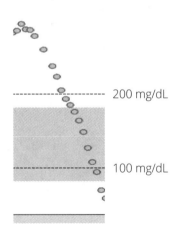

200 mg/dL

100 mg/dL

Blood glucose lows and acceleration downward. If the blood glucose is low and leveling off, the standard amount of carbohydrate should work fine (see next image).

SECRET STRATEGY #14

Know when to say when! When assisting someone who is experiencing hypoglycemia, resist the urge to over-treat. Hypoglycemia can stimulate hunger in a *big* way. The person experiencing the low may keep asking for more and more food, but this

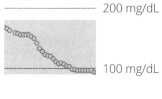

200 mg/dL

100 mg/dL

Blood glucose is mildly low but leveling off. The shaded area is the blood glucose target zone of 80–170 mg/dL.

will not help raise blood glucose any faster. Over-treating with food will likely produce a significantly high blood glucose within the next couple of hours.

Choosing the Best Treatment for Hypoglycemia

Not all carbs are created equal. Some will raise the blood glucose quickly, while others will take their sweet time (excuse the play on words). When treating a low, choose a food that will raise it as quickly as possible, and check the labels for the exact serving size and grams of carbohydrate. Examples include:

➤ Glucose tablets

➤ Candies made with dextrose (including SweetTARTS, Smarties, Spree, AirHeads, Runts, and Nerds)

➤ Sport drinks

➤ Orange or grape juice

➤ Cereal

➤ Pretzels/crackers

➤ Jelly beans

➤ Vanilla wafers

➤ Graham crackers

Foods that contain a great deal of fat or fiber are going to take much longer to raise blood glucose and should only be used as a last resort. Even some "healthy" foods such as milk and whole fruit can take quite a while to work.

It usually takes 10–15 minutes for rapid-acting carbohydrates to *start* raising the blood glucose and 30–60 minutes for them to work completely. So be patient! Many people over-treat their lows and wind up very, very high as a result. Check blood glucose 15–20 minutes after treating the low. If it has not risen above 70 mg/dL, go ahead and treat again. If it is above 70 mg/dL, all should be fine.

FACTOID #21

CGM systems tend to produce false low readings for 30–60 minutes after a low has been treated. There is a prolonged lag time when in the state of hypoglycemia. Use fingerstick readings to confirm that the blood glucose has returned to a safe level.

By the way, it is not necessary to consume protein or complex/slowly digesting carbs after treating a low. As long as the blood glucose has returned to a safe level after treatment, there is no reason to expect it to drop again suddenly. In fact, the blood glucose may continue to climb for a few hours because of a hormonal "rebound." However, be on the lookout for low blood glucose later in the day, or even the next day. A person's risk of hypoglycemia increases modestly for 24 hours after each low glucose episode.

Treating Severe Low Glucose Levels
Severe hypoglycemia, when a person is unwilling or unable to consciously swallow food, must be treated differently than mild and moderate low episodes. It is dangerous to put any kind of food into the mouth of individuals having a severe low. They could choke on the food and suffocate, or they could instinctively bite down and take the fingers off the person trying to feed them.

SECRET STRATEGY #15

Never force food into the mouth of someone who is unconscious or uncooperative.

There are two things, and only two things, you should do to help someone having a severe low blood glucose: call for emergency help and administer an injection of glucagon. It is important to deal with severe hypoglycemia as quickly as possible to avoid severe injuries (from falls or seizures), coma, permanent neurological damage, and even death.

Glucagon (or Glucagen) is not sugar. It is a hormone that raises blood glucose by stimulating the liver to release its stored-up sugar into the bloodstream. It will usually work in 10–20 minutes. Glucagon is a prescription item that comes in a kit containing a large fluid-filled syringe, a small vial with the glucagon hormone in powder form, and instructions written in a seemingly foreign language. The kits have an expiration date, but they are usually good for 6–12 months past the expiration date as long as they have been stored properly at room temperature. We recommend saving expired kits so that you can practice with them (on a pillow or foam ball, not your loved ones!).

Glucagon Kit

The procedure for administering glucagon is as follows:

1. Call 9-1-1. Have paramedics on the way in case the glucagon injection fails to work.

2. Pull the cap off the syringe and flip the cap off the vial.

3. Inject all of the fluid into the vial.

4. Remove the syringe from the vial. Keep pressure on the plunger to make sure air does not escape from the vial.

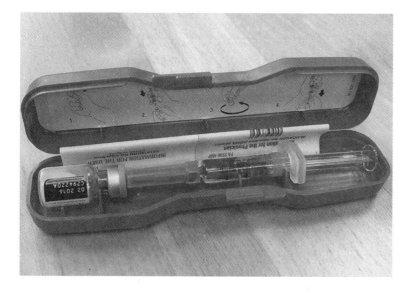

5. Shake or swirl the vial gently until the fluid is evenly mixed (no clumps) and mostly clear.

6. With the vial held upside down, reinsert the tip of the needle into the vial. (Do *not* put the whole needle in; you will draw in air accidentally!)

7. Draw the fluid into the syringe. For very small children (under age 6), it is fine to only draw about half of the fluid into the syringe. For older children and adults, draw in the majority of the fluid.

8. Insert the needle straight (not at an angle) into a muscle such as the thigh or shoulder. Inject the full contents of the syringe.

9. Remove the syringe and apply a tissue to suppress any bleeding.

10. Turn the victim onto his or her side to prevent choking (in case vomiting occurs).

Your loved one should regain consciousness in 10–20 minutes. If he or she does not, wait for paramedics to arrive. Contact your health care team to troubleshoot and work on a plan for preventing severe lows from happening again.

Glucagon is 100% the responsibility of you, the support person. Make sure you have a prescription for it and have at least one kit on hand at all times. Plan to replace it yearly, or right away if you must use it. Take it with you when you travel, and be prepared to use it when needed.

Glucagon readiness checklist:

➤ Have prescription

➤ Have kit on hand

➤ Be trained on use

➤ Be mentally prepared to use in an emergency

Is There a Way to Prevent Hypoglycemia?

Recognize that just about everyone who takes insulin experiences low blood glucose from time to time. An occasional bout of hypoglycemia is no reason to panic. However, if the low levels are severe or become a pattern (occurring at about the same time of day on a semi-regular basis), talk to your health care team about possible solutions. In addition to daily management approaches, new technologies such as CGMs (which can warn users before a low takes place) and hybrid closed-loop insulin pumps (which stop insulin delivery automatically if a low is anticipated) are effective tools for helping to prevent hypoglycemia. Even if having occasional lows, try to troubleshoot what is causing the hypoglycemia: What is the likely cause, and how can a repeat occurrence be avoided? You may find it helpful to refer to the "usual suspects" list on page 166 in Chapter 6.

While preventing hypoglycemia is a worthwhile endeavor, be careful not to go to extremes. Some caregivers become obsessed about preventing hypoglycemia, fearing that it will lead to death. While it is true that people have died as a result of hypoglycemia (either from getting into serious accidents or simply failing to recover from a severe/prolonged low), the risk of this happening is less than the chance of being run over by a bus. We need to take *reasonable* precautions to prevent both, but we can't allow fear to dominate our thinking. In clinical practice, we have seen many patients, young and old, whose families obsess so much over hypoglycemia that they run their blood glucose levels dangerously high all the time. You wouldn't stay inside all the time to avoid being hit by that bus, so don't let an irrational fear of lows interfere with a healthy approach to diabetes management.

Managing High Blood Glucose Levels

The topic of managing high blood glucose integrates many of the lessons and principles we've discussed so far. First, let's get the terminology right. The word "high" is vague and, in some cases, judgmental. This word can also lead to false conclusions in conversation: "She stayed home from work today because she was really high." Get the idea? Let's apply a "word swap" like we discussed in Chapter 4. Henceforth, we'll refer to it as "above-target." This term is more objective and only describes the blood glucose, not the person.

Of course, it would be helpful to know what the target is! This is a discussion for you to have with your partner and/or his or her health care provider. Remember, target ranges should be realistic (acceptable) and not "perfect." This is different from the specific number that we aim for when calculating correction doses of insulin. For example, in young children, we often set the target range at 80–200 mg/dL. In older children, 70–180 mg/dL is commonly acceptable. For adults with type 1 diabetes, 70–160 mg/dL is a typical range, and the goal during pregnancy is usually 60–140 mg/dL. For people with type 2 diabetes who are not taking mealtime insulin, 70–120 or 80–140 mg/dL are common premeal targets.

Next, let's consider how you found out your loved one's blood glucose is above target. As a caregiver, it may be your role to obtain this information directly (via a meter's memory, shared CGM data, or inspection of a logbook). After all, you probably need this information for determining insulin doses and to keep your loved one safe. But as a support person, there are really only two ways you should know that a blood glucose is above target: *1)* you recognize symptoms in your partner (excess thirst/urination, lethargy, irritability) and inquire about his or her status or *2)* he or she offers up this information freely and without coercion. And if you're relying on symptoms, try to inquire in a nonjudgmental way—in a way that allows your partner to volunteer the information. "I noticed you're running to the bathroom a lot more than usual. Is everything OK?" is a much better approach than "You're peeing constantly. You're blood glucose is high again, isn't it?"

Once you've determined (or have been informed) that your loved one's blood glucose is elevated, consider how he or she is probably feeling. Empathy goes a long way toward helping in a positive, constructive manner. Your loved one is probably thirsty, so offer to get something to drink. Or better yet, just bring something to drink and say, "I thought you might like this." Your loved one's mind may be a bit cloudy, so don't ask to perform any complex mental tasks. Better yet, take some mental work off of his or her plate. Your loved one's energy level is likely to be low, so it's not a good time to mow the lawn or perform any heavy exercise. But knowing how physical activity can improve the situation, you might ask him or her to take a relaxing walk with you, or take a pet for a walk. And given that moods can be a bit out of kilter, try to be understanding if things are said that normally wouldn't be. And by all means, choose another time to address issues that can be a source of conflict.

Of course, desperate times call for desperate measures. Severely elevated blood glucose levels, or readings that stay above target for prolonged periods of time, may merit a discussion with your partner. But remember to express yourself from the perspective of someone who cares, and not someone who is judging. "Honey, all these elevated readings have got to be taking a toll on you. Maybe we can give your diabetes educator a call" comes across much better than "No wonder you're high all the time. You never exercise and you're eating constantly!" The words you choose can make a world of difference.

KEY POINTS

> ➤ Hypoglycemia is classified as "mild," "moderate," and "severe."

> ➤ Mild and moderate lows should be treated with appropriate amounts of rapid-acting carbohydrate.

> ➤ Unconscious/unresponsive lows should not be treated with food, but with glucagon and, if necessary, emergency medical services.

> ➤ Over-treating lows and taking extreme measures to avoid lows tend to be counterproductive.

> ➤ Patterns of hypoglycemia and hyperglycemia usually warrant a change in the management approach.

> ➤ Be diplomatic in the way you find out about your partner's high readings and how you address them.

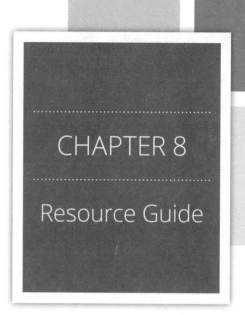

The American Diabetes Association (ADA) provides an excellent online dictionary of common diabetes terms. This dictionary can help you learn the new language of diabetes and diabetes management and can help you understand the information coming from health care providers and other resources: http://www.diabetes.org/diabetes-basics/common-terms.

Technologies, Tools, and Apps

The intersection of technology and medicine has brought many exciting improvements to diabetes management. We have new ways to track, treat, and monitor various aspects of diabetes management. Many of these advances are true game-changers in improving our ability to effectively manage diabetes and improve health outcomes.

However, we all might be misled by the dazzle of blood glucose readings showing up on phones and watches, meters that talk, pumps replacing injections, and apps that log and highlight blood glucose patterns with game-like characters. What gets lost in the technological glow is the awareness that the basic principles of diabetes management remain the same today as they did 30 years ago. The brutal reality is that technology has not been able to substantially reduce the burden of living with and managing diabetes. In some ways, the wave of new technology has brought increased management requirements and expectations.

The trade-off is clear: diabetes management before technological advances (insulin once a day, no carb counting, checking blood glucose only at the doctor's office, etc.) required less work on a day-to-day basis, but diabetes-related complications were much more likely. Now, with better knowledge and tools, we see fewer complications, but the daily burden of managing all these tools and taking action on the information they provide is much greater. Simply put, people can live healthier lives with diabetes today than they could 20 years ago, but it comes with a high investment of time and money to do so.

Therefore, while this section is about highlighting technologies that make us "better" at diabetes management, it also highlights the need to continue to push research and industry to achieve advances that not only improve health outcomes, but also reduce the human burden and effort it takes to apply, interpret, and manage these advances.

That said, let's get back to the gadgets, tools, and technologies that are sweeping the diabetes scene! The number of apps and online communities is ever-growing. And the good news is that many of the better ones are free! We've listed below some of our favorite programs and apps.

GoMeal: Links with Fitbit to integrate food consumed with activity and calories burned.

SparkPeople: Weight loss website and app that has a great recipe calculator to determine carbs/fat/calories/protein for homemade recipes. The carb feature on this is key to making it easier for people using the carb-counting method to eat homemade rather than packaged foods.

Livongo: Cellular-enabled meter that provides real-time treatment recommendations to the meter, unlimited test strips, and 24/7 access to certified diabetes educators.

MySugr and MySugr, Jr: Brings some fun and compassion to diabetes tracking.

Pebble or Apple Watch: Receive blood glucose data on a watch.

Dexcom Share and Dexcom Mobile: Share real-time CGM data with others.

HealthyOut: Identifies healthier choices when dining out at chain restaurants. Choices are based on eating preferences, e.g., low carb, paleo, low fat. There's even an option for "not salad."

Calorie King: The original carb/calorie index, for both name-brand items and nonpackaged items.

Headspace: Easy, relatable way to get started with meditation for stress management. They even have a version specifically for kids.

Connected or Smart Meters: Ask your insurance provider which smart meter and strips they will cover. Few people are able (or willing) to write down every blood glucose reading, meal, activity, and insulin/medication dose. Meters that capture your data and remove the need for manual recordkeeping greatly improve your (and your doctor's) ability to make the right adjustments. You can also ask your doctor to write a letter of medical necessity for a smart meter/ strips if your insurance doesn't cover one.

My Fitness Pal: Can be used by people with or without diabetes. It provides a large database of foods and provides a breakdown of the food content. It also has easy trackers for exercise and weight.

....

Professional Resources

We've all heard the saying, "It takes a village to raise a child." Well, it also takes a team of experts to help someone living with diabetes manage successfully.

Surrounding your loved one with a quality health care team is like putting together a winning baseball team. Each player has a role, yet all should work together for the ultimate goal: in this case, the well-being of your loved one. There may be times when you have to trade players, but that's OK. While there is value to continuity, it can also be beneficial to get a fresh perspective from time to time. And of course, if someone is not doing the job to your satisfaction, you have every right to fire that person and bring in someone new.

As complex as diabetes management can be, many people benefit from working with a "multidisciplinary team" of health care experts. The American Diabetes Association maintains a current list of "recognized diabetes self-management programs," most of which feature a group of diabetes care experts with diverse expertise. Although there are many quality providers not included on the list, the programs on the list have all been recognized by the American Diabetes Association for meeting national standards for diabetes education and treatment. For an updated list, go to http://professional. diabetes.org/erp_list, or call 800-342-2383.

Look for the following to create your own all-star team of diabetes consultants:

Certified diabetes educator (CDE): A CDE is often a nurse or dietitian, but it can also be a pharmacist, exercise physiologist, physician, mental health counselor, or anyone in the health care field with advanced training in diabetes management. Your CDE should be able to coach you and your loved one through the complexities of living day-to-day with diabetes. To locate a CDE in your area, visit the

American Association of Diabetes Educators CDE network at http://www.diabeteseducator.org/DiabetesEducation/Find.html.

Physician (MD or DO): Different physicians have different levels of expertise in treating diabetes. **Endocrinologists** typically have the most experience and skill in diabetes care. Look for endocrinologists who are board certified; this ensures that they receive continuing education and are updated on the latest treatment methods. To find a board-certified physician, visit the American Board of Medical Specialties website, www.abms.org. Internal medicine doctors (**internists**) usually treat a variety of chronic health conditions. Some have a great deal of expertise in treating diabetes. Most **general practitioners** (family doctors) and **nurse practitioners** have a basic understanding of how to manage diabetes, but they also can make sure that you receive all the necessary screenings and treatments for other health problems related to diabetes (called *comorbidities).*

Registered dietitian nutritionist (RD or RDN): Given the major role that food plays in living healthy with diabetes, it pays to have a nutrition expert in your corner. An RD or RDN can help you with carb counting, weight control, sports nutrition, alcohol safety, and specialized meal planning. To find an RD or RDN who specializes in diabetes, contact the Academy of Nutrition and Dietetics at 800-877-1600 or visit www.eatright.org/public (click on the "find an expert" icon).

Mental health counselor: With all the pressure placed on people with diabetes and their loved ones, a social worker, psychologist, or psychiatrist can be a valuable member of your health care team. Mental health professionals can help with issues such as stress, depression, eating disorders, sleep disturbances, obsessive/compulsive behaviors, anxieties, relationship difficulties, financial hardship, and job discrimination. Don't hesitate to ask your primary physician for a referral to a mental health professional if the need arises.

National Association of Social Workers is a good resource, too: https://www.helppro.com/nasw/BasicSearch.aspx.

An exercise specialist: Despite its many benefits, exercise can be challenging for people with diabetes because of blood glucose control issues and other health problems. An exercise physiologist is a health professional who can help you design an exercise plan, formulate strategies to prevent hypoglycemia, manage blood glucose levels during sports/competitive activities, and reduce your risk for injuries and other complications. Look for an exercise physiologist who is also a certified diabetes educator (CDE).

Specialists: Given the many bodily systems that are affected by diabetes, your loved one's health care team may need to include a few other specialists. These might include:

➤ Podiatrist (for prevention and treatment of foot problems)

➤ Ophthalmologist (for routine eye exams and treatment of eye disorders)

➤ Dentist (for ongoing tooth/gum care and treatment of periodontal disease)

➤ Nephrologist (for treatment of kidney disease)

➤ Neurologist (for treatment of nerve disorders)

➤ Cardiologist or vascular surgeon (for treatment of blood vessel diseases)

Personal Resources

Living with diabetes can be a frustrating, and sometimes frightening, experience for you and your loved one. At times, it can also make you feel very alone.

If you have ever felt the need to reach out to someone who understands how you feel (someone who has *been there*), support networks may be just the answer. Even if you don't feel the need to receive support yourself, the act of giving support to others can be very therapeutic.

SECRET STRATEGY #16

"A man's gotta know his limitations."

– Dirty Harry Callahan

For an in-person type of support group, a good place to start is your local hospital or diabetes treatment center. If there is a diabetes association office near you, check there for a listing of support groups in your area. If nothing exists near you, or if what exists fails to meet your needs, consider starting a group of your own. Post flyers at doctors' offices, and let your local ADA and Juvenile Diabetes Research Foundation chapters know so that they can share the information with their members.

If face-to-face groups are not feasible, consider participating in (or starting) an online community or group. Although information derived from online groups may not always be 100% accurate, you can still gain an emotional lift from conversing with other people facing similar challenges.

Resources are not limited to mutual support–type programs. There is also an assortment of clinical support, associations, media/publications, government entities, books, product manufacturers, and mail-order suppliers ready to serve you. Below is a list of some of the resources we've found to be highly useful.

Helpful Personal Resources

To find a dietitian, contact the Academy of Nutrition and Dietetics at 800-877-1600 or visit www.eatright.org/public (click on the "find an expert" icon).

To locate a diabetes educator, visit the American Association of Diabetes Educators at http://www.diabeteseducator. org/DiabetesEducation/Find.html.

For unlimited resources for kids and parents, visit www. childrenwithdiabetes.com.

For parents of kids with diabetes, visit www.parenting diabetickids.com.

To reach a community of people touched by diabetes, run by the Diabetes Hands Foundation, visit www.tudiabetes.org.

For information on the ups and downs of life with a child with diabetes, visit http://www.d-mom.com.

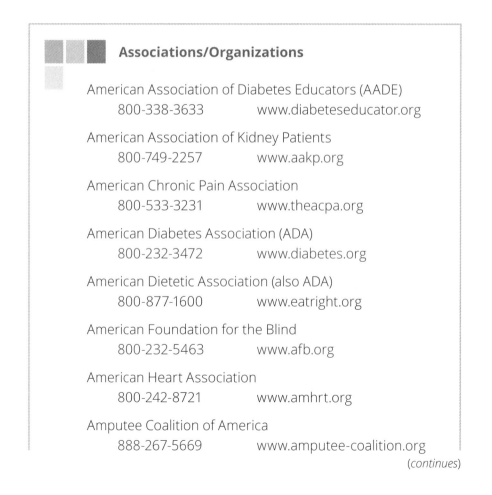

Associations/Organizations

American Association of Diabetes Educators (AADE)
    800-338-3633   www.diabeteseducator.org

American Association of Kidney Patients
    800-749-2257   www.aakp.org

American Chronic Pain Association
    800-533-3231   www.theacpa.org

American Diabetes Association (ADA)
    800-232-3472   www.diabetes.org

American Dietetic Association (also ADA)
    800-877-1600   www.eatright.org

American Foundation for the Blind
    800-232-5463   www.afb.org

American Heart Association
    800-242-8721   www.amhrt.org

Amputee Coalition of America
    888-267-5669   www.amputee-coalition.org

(*continues*)

Associations/Organizations (*Continued*)

Celiac Society
> 504-305-2968   www.celiacsociety.com

Celiac Sprue Association/USA
> 402-558-0600   www.csaceliacs.org

Diabetes Camping Association (DCA)
> 256-883-2556   www.diabetescamps.org

Friends With Diabetes (Jewish)
> 845-352-7532   www.friendswithdiabetes.org

International Association for Medical Assistance
to Travelers (IAMAT)
> 716-754-4883   www.iamat.org

Gluten Intolerance Group of North America
> 206-246-6652   www.gluten.net

Jewish Diabetes Association (JDA)
> 718-787-4532   www.jewishdiabetes.org

Juvenile Diabetes Research Foundation (JDRF)
> 800-533-2873   www.jdrf.org

National Center on Physical Activity and Disability
> 800-900-8086   www.ncpad.org

National Federation of the Blind Materials
Resource Center
> 410-659-9314   www.nfb.org

National Kidney Foundation
> 800-622-9010   www.kidney.org

National Institute of Dental and Craniofacial Research
> 301-402-7364   www.nidcr.nih.gov

(*continues*)

Associations/Organizations (*Continued*)

National Institute of Diabetes and Digestive
and Kidney Diseases
    301-496-3583   www.niddk.nih.gov

National Library Service for the Blind
and Physically Handicapped
    800-424-8567

Neuropathy Association
    800-247-6968   www.neuropathy.org

National Diabetes Education Program
    800-GET-LEVEL   www.niddk.nih.gov/health/
                          diabetes/ndep/ndep.htm

National Diabetes Information Clearinghouse
    800-860-8747   www.niddk.nih.gov/health/
                          diabetes/ndc.htmm
    301-496-4261   www.nih.gov

Taking Control of Your Diabetes (TCOYD)
    800-998-2693   www.tcoyd.org

Type 1 Diabetes TrialNet
    800-425-8361   http://www.diabetestrialnet.org

Financial Resources

Medicare is a government-sponsored program for people over age 65 as well as younger people with serious health problems such as kidney failure. Medicare covers blood glucose monitors, test strips, lancets, insulin pumps/supplies, therapeutic shoes, glaucoma screenings, flu and pneumonia vaccines, and limited counseling by some registered dietitians and certified diabetes educators. Medicare Part D provides prescription drug benefits for items such as insulin and oral diabetes medications. For eligibility information, call the Centers for Medicare & Medicaid Services at 1-800-633-4227, or visit www.medicare.gov.

Medicaid is a health assistance program sponsored by each individual state. Eligibility is based on your income level. Medicaid recipients may qualify for full or partial coverage for select types of diabetes medications and blood glucose monitors/strips. For information, contact the Department of Human Services in the "government" pages of your phone book.

The **Children's Health Insurance Program**, or **CHIP**, is provided by each state. It is for children whose families earn too much to qualify for Medicaid but too little to afford private health insurance. For information, call 877-543-7669, or visit www.insurekidsnow.gov.

The Bureau of Primary Health Care (also called the Hill-Burton Program) offers professional medical care regardless of insurance status or ability to pay. For a directory of local primary health care centers, call 800-400-2742 or visit www.bphc.hrsa.gov.

The VA (Department of Veterans Affairs) runs hospitals and clinics for veterans who need treatment for service-related ailments and/or financial aid. To find out more about VA health benefits, call 800-827-1000 or visit www.va.gov.

WIC (Women, Infants, and Children) can assist women and children with diabetes who need nutritional help. Healthy eating is an essential component of diabetes self-care. Women with preexisting diabetes who become pregnant, as well as women who develop gestational diabetes, may be eligible for assistance with grocery costs if certain criteria are met. For more information, call the WIC headquarters at 703-305-2746 or visit www.fns.usda.gov/wic.

Blink Health is a free app that gives access to discounts on diabetes and other types of medications. Visit www. blinkhealth.com for more information.

People who have no prescription coverage and are not eligible for Medicare may be able to obtain a free **Together Rx Access Card.** Using the card can save you 25–40% on a select list of brand-name and generic drugs/supplies (including insulin, oral diabetes medications, meters, and test strips). For qualification information and a list of covered drugs, call 800-444-4106 or visit www.togetherrxaccess.com.

Rx Assist provides a comprehensive database of pharmaceutical assistance programs.

Visit www.rxassist.org.

Needy Meds has information on pharmaceutical and health care assistance programs at www.needymeds.org.

Partnership for Prescription Assistance helps qualifying patients without prescription drug coverage get the medicines they need for free or nearly free. Visit www.pparx.org.

RxHope is a web-based resource that acts as a facilitator in helping people get their medications for free or for a small copayment. Visit www.rxhope.com or call 877-267-0517.

BenefitsCheckUp® is a service of the National Council on Aging that has information on benefits programs for seniors with limited income and resources. Seniors can search for programs that help them pay for prescription drugs as well as health care, rent, utilities, and other needs. Visit www. benefitscheckup.org.

Lilly Cares is a patient assistance program for users of Eli Lilly insulin and other medications. Free insulin is provided by way of coupons supplied to your physician. Lilly Cares is open to legal U.S. residents who fail to qualify for government-sponsored programs, do not have private insurance, and fall below a certain income level. For more information, call 800-545-6962 or visit www.lillycares.com.

Novo Nordisk offers a Patient Assistance Program that provides free insulin, pen needles, and glucagon kits for people who fail to qualify for government-sponsored programs, do not have private insurance, and fall below a certain income level. For more information, call 866-310-7549 or visit www.novonordisk-us.com.

Sanofi-Aventis Pharmaceuticals also offers a Patient Assistance Program that provides free insulin to people who fail to qualify for government-sponsored programs, do not have private insurance, and fall below a certain income level. For more information, call 800-221-4025 or visit www.sanofi.us.

Glucose Test Strip manufacturers often provide copay cards for users of their blood glucose meters. The copay cards either reduce or eliminate copays associated with test strip purchases. There are usually no income or insurance eligibility limits. For details, call the toll-free number on the back of your glucose meter.

In the U.S., each state has its own **Attorney General's Office** whose job is to enforce laws and regulations of that particular state. Because most health care standards are enacted and governed by each state, the Attorney General's Office can come to your aid if you feel that you are being dealt with unfairly by your health insurance, health care providers, pharmaceutical company, or a medical device manufacturer. Check in the white pages of your phone book, or search online for the Attorney General's Office for your particular state.

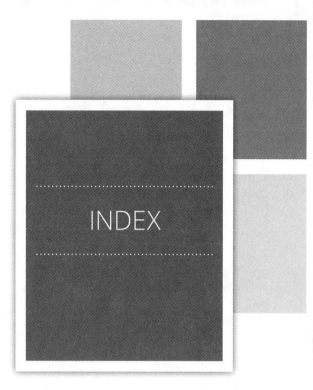

INDEX

Note: page numbers in **bold** refer to in-depth discussions.